M000234327

8-2001

Bypass

Bypass

a memoir

Joseph A. Amato

PURDUE UNIVERSITY PRESS
West Lafayette, Indiana

Design and composition by inari

Library of Congress Cataloging-in-Publication Data

Amato, Joseph Anthony.
    Bypass : a memoir / by Joseph A. Amato ; forewords by
Leon Rappoport and Lyle Joyce.
        p.   cm.
    ISBN 1-55753-176-5 (alk. paper)
    1. Amato, Joseph Anthony—Health. 2. Coronary artery
bypass—Patients—United States—Biography. I. Title.
    RD598.35.C67 A45 2000
    362.1'97412'0092—dc21

                                            00-008404

Contents

Rehabilitation

To Cathy
My Second Heart

"All that I can say is that in more ways than one my heart
has been touched, and I am not, and shall never be, quite the
same person."

Joseph Epstein, "Taking the Bypass"
The New Yorker (April 12, 1999)

Foreword

Some Reflections on Amato's Bypass

Leon Rappoport

The profound truism that has already become a cliché of our postmodern era is that everything is connected to everything else. Chaos theorists refer to this as the "butterfly effect": let a butterfly fall to earth and the whole world system is definitely altered. The world of Joe Amato was definitely altered when, like a butterfly in distress, his heart lost its lifelong rhythm and began a fluttering struggle to regain it.

If this book was simply the story of how an apparently ordinary middle-aged college professor experienced his heart condition and subsequent bypass surgery, it might be worth reading as a matter of curiosity, or perhaps as a cautionary tale and forewarning to all of us who have so far escaped the chest pains and breathing difficulties that first brought Joe to his physician's office. And if the social-emotional events revealed as he found himself gradually reduced to the status of just one more anonymous cardiac "case" lack the imperative drama of, say, a "live from the battlefield" report by Peter Arnett, it does have its remarkable moments. The issue is, after all, life or death. And it is no small matter either when the newly anonymous patient finds that his life depends upon the acquiescence to the indignities that come from being carefully tested and measured in order to assure a good fit into the high tech, procrustean bed of modern medicine.

But Joe Amato is NOT your ordinary middle-aged college professor (although he has learned to enjoy passing for one). He did not go quietly into that procrustean bed, and the book tells far more than the story of his heart condition. On the contrary, as any reader will quickly perceive, inside the prosaic professor there dwells a near-demonic intelligence suffused with a Faustian passion for life! These qualities make him a wonderfully stimulating author—like any good Catholic intellectual, he is always ready to argue with God or the Devil—but, as the medics say, a difficult patient. Witness, for example, his tears of rage and sadness following routine diagnostic procedures, his vision of an angiogram as a snake being slowly wiggled into his heart, and the portrait of his heart surgeon as a high priest presiding over the blood sacrifice rituals of the operating theater. Moreover, although the heart condition serves as the skeletal theme of the narrative, the larger story fleshed out on this theme is nothing less than a critical reintegration and meditation upon his life history.

Perhaps I am biased from too many years working in the field of life span development and psychobiography, but it seems to me that what makes this book exceptional is the unusually candid, multi-dimensional view it provides of a quintessentially American life. In many ways, the story emerging from the flashbacks to childhood, youth, the gropings toward an adult identity and its ultimate achievement, is an archetype of the American Dream: the streetwise boy from a working-class Italian-American family in Detroit who works his way up to the Good Life of a respected scholar-professor.

Another cliché? In outline, yes, but in substance, no, because Amato's narrative is informed throughout by a series of critical internal dialogues; unsparing conversations with himself that unveil the uniquely ambivalent nature of the American Dream. What it gives with one hand, it takes away with the other; there is no free lunch; no gain without pain. Thus, on a visit back to the Detroit of his childhood he discovers — of course — that is had virtually disappeared. The successful middle-aged American in the shadow of life-threatening disease seeks to make peace with the past that he once enthusiastically left behind him, but finds mainly . . . emptiness, and a few artifacts sufficient to stimulate memories. Yet it is from his interrogation of those memories — of his failure to fight a local bully who called him "Dago"; of the girl he loved at age fourteen; of the country club where he worked as a caddie; and of the hardworking, loving but distant father who in the end remained a mystery to him — that he can begin to tie the meaning of his life to that of his parents and grandparents, his wife, children, and their children. In short, what we have here, finally, is an account of how one extraordinary scholar could put his own life up on the board for examination and work through it to a point of transcendence and acceptance. The transcendence is what Christians call "agape" (Look it up!), and Zen Buddhists call "going beyond the self": a recognition of self as inseparable from the larger, unending flow of existential being. Does this eliminate fear of death, bring peace of mind, saintly wisdom and forbearance? Hell no! Not for most Zen masters and certainly not for Amato. But it does bring him acceptance, no small thing, and on good days, even a bit of grace.

It shows up beautifully at the end of the book when, after recovering from the surgery only to be thrust back again to his physicians because of side effects from certain medications, he is safely home for Christmas:

> I watched the pope bless the people in Vatican Square on Christmas morning, and read Matthew's and Luke's nativity accounts. I thought of Luther's confession: I cannot believe in Christ as I should . . . . [T]he "old donkey" in me won't have it . . . . In my heart it is just as bad as it is in the world.

Amato's closing to his convalescence, though, is a perfect realization of what life span psychologists call "ego integrity":

> I believed that on some terms or other I would go on. Perhaps God wanted to soften me more, and further wring the child out of the man. In any case, as long as I had these legs, I would continue to skate—I would still glide across this dark ice.

Foreword

Lyle Joyce

With heart disease as the number one killer in America, coronary artery bypass surgery has become a common surgical procedure. Even though technology and development have considerably lowered the risk factor, it is still a life and death operation. Joe Amato has articulated the fears each patient goes through before and during heart surgery. He has given insight into the physical, emotional, and spiritual struggles that a patient faces when confronted with the possibility of death. He notes that it is a time to reflect on the past, fear the future, and have one's faith either strengthened or weakened.

For several hours a team of anesthesiologists, perfusionists, nurses, a first assistant, and I captained an array of machines and instruments to repair Joseph Amato's heart. I did an operation I had performed thousands of times before in my previous twenty-five years as a surgeon.

The bypass surgery went smoothly. No unexpected problems were discovered when we opened Joe's chest. As the angiogram had suggested, we faced a straightforward bypass. In addition to using veins from his leg for grafts, we were able to redirect the internal mammary artery, attaching it to two arteries on the left side of the heart to supplement blood supply to the blocked vessels.

Right from the start, Amato's prognosis was good. He had no previous heart damage. He was relatively young—in his mid-fifties. On the basis of an extended telephone conversation with him months before the operation and from a meeting with him on the day of surgery, I judged Amato to be determined and full of vitality. Displaying neither defeat nor hopeless resignation, his intent in having the operation was to get on with his busy life. He had been referred to me by his doctor in Marshall, Minnesota, and he was adamant that no one else but me should do his surgery.

Until I read his book, I had no idea of the internal journey Amato had traveled during his heart bypass experience. Amato transformed the operation—breaking open his chest, packing his heart in ice, and providing his heart with a new supply of blood—into a whole constellation of metaphors around which he reorganized the meaning of life.

For a few hours, our surgical team directed our attention to repairing the organ before us. In our hands, Amato's heart was yet another pump, a truly amazing and life-giving engine, that had to be mechanically repaired. The successful repair job was rewarded with a patient who left the hospital in much better physical health. Another reward is this compelling book about a patient's trip to and from bypass surgery. This book has a message not only about the personal history of Amato, but also about the history of medicine.

In the author's lifetime, physicians have gone from the "practice of medicine" to being controlled by the impersonal "medical system" of a highly technical, scientific approach to patient care. When Amato was a child in the 1940s and 1950s, his physician had little to offer him in the way of complex scientific tests and sophisticated therapeutic modalities. In many instances, the physician's personal bedside manner was as critical as the medicines he distributed and the operations he performed. The confidence the patient had to get through a surgical procedure or recover from an illness was largely dependent on trust in his or her physician.

Amato's story reminds us that despite the metamorphoses of medical practice, the patient's personal and emotional needs have not changed. What has changed is the process by which a physical illness is diagnosed and treated. The diagnosis is made with the assistance of many highly technical tests and procedures, and the treatment is even more dependent on specialized, expensive, technical equipment. The potential for success is now primarily measured by the results of the technical tests and procedures. A physician's ability to control the critical relationship between physician and patient has lessened considerably. Today the doctor is more and more controlled by the medical system.

Amato reveals his frustration about this in his book. He worries about the doctor-patient relationship being disrupted when a healthcare provider negotiates a new contract with another system that excludes the patient's current doctor. There is also the threat of changing coverage in an insurance program.

Having enjoyed being a part of the technological advancements in the treatment of heart disease, I am confident that life as a whole is better with the addition of such things as heart catheterizations, angioplasties, heart-lung machines, and artificial hearts. However, the healthcare system has become more fragmented with the addition of each of these innovations in diagnosis and therapy. Medicine's challenge now is to restore the best of both worlds. Medicine must put patients' needs first. The heart hospital of the future should provide a holistic healing experience for the patient and the patient's family.

I want to thank the author, my patient, for asking me to write this foreword. I have learned from him, and I am sure all who read this book will benefit from his insights into the journey of bypass surgery.

Bypass

Diagnosis

My heart problem was first diagnosed by a stress test in 1988. After a week of experiencing difficulty in breathing on my after-lunch walks and tightness in my chest on one of my after-supper solitary golf rounds, with my wife's encouragement, I went to the doctor.

Upon hearing of my symptoms, which also included more burping than usual, our family doctor, Doctor Kaczrowski (whom I call "Kacz"), ordered a blood test and stress test. One afternoon a week later I returned home from the doctor and, doing what I hadn't done since I was a boy, burst into tears. My tears were brief and hot and profuse. I told my wife that I wasn't depressed or overwhelmed by my condition but was simply crying for my youth and the good health that I had now clearly lost.

Although I had been overweight by forty or fifty pounds (210 instead of a more desirable 170 or 160) since I had been married, I was in good shape, and I always felt healthy. I ate and drank pretty much at will. I never got stomachaches or headaches. Twenty-five years of smoking, which I quit at age thirty-seven, had not taken away my lungs: I skated, golfed, played racquetball, rode a bike, and played goalie on a college broomball team, which one year won our small city league. Yet now, a few symptoms and one diagnosis had turned my world upside down.

In my meeting with Kacz I was told within a matter of a few sentences that I had both adult diabetes and blockage in my heart. C. Paul Martin, our clinic's internist who ran the treadmill stress test, suspected blockage in at least two vessels. It was confirmed by another colleague, "Olie" Odland, at the local clinic. Odland, whose expertise in cardiology was supplemented and given the voice of authenticity by his own recent heart attack and bypass, concluded that I was an asymptomatic case. He told me I suffered silent aschemia (a word whose mixture of *s* and *e* sounds alone were enough to scare me without knowing its exact meaning). It meant that I could suffer, as did Odland, a heart attack without warning. Not hesitant in expressing his opinion, Odland thought I should have immediate surgery. He even recommended his surgeon, Lyle Joyce of Abbott Northwestern, as the best in the state. Kacz concurred with Martin's and Odland's diagnoses. He told me to arrange an angiogram at the Minneapolis Heart Institute at Abbott Northwestern as soon as possible.

He explained what an angiogram was: The surgery team would enter my body through an artery in my groin. Then they would thread a small camera up the artery into the arteries of my heart in order to determine the extent of arterial blockage. If one or several of my arteries were significantly blocked, which would threaten the oxygen supply to my heart, they would recommend a bypass.

I don't know whether the metaphor of a snake crawling through my heart reached my consciousness at the time, but I do know the idea of them entering into that vital organ filled me with fear and revulsion. But they assured me the operation was safe: It was, Kacz said, about as dangerous as driving from Minneapolis to Chicago. I reflected on traffic conditions I had encountered during family trips from Minnesota to Detroit around Chicago. Not asking whether it would be rush hour, which we always tried to avoid, I agreed without much fuss to the angiogram. My wife (a nurse) and I agreed. We entered into a covenanted fiction, as husbands and wives do on so many matters great and small, that the angiogram was simply a routine medical procedure.

A week later, my sister-in-law, who was visiting us from Virginia and wishing to see the Twin Cities, and I started out on a three-hour car trip from my house in Marshall, in southwestern Minnesota, to Abbott Northwestern. I kept the conversation away from my heart as much as I could and clung to the idea that the angiogram was routine. She cooperated in finding other things to talk about, knowing as well as I that tomorrow I would receive information that might change my whole life.

The day of the angiogram didn't start well. I had barely sat down in the small waiting room when, from behind the doors to the pre-operation room, an old friend entered. Lil was sobbing, and I held her hand for half an hour or so as she waited for the outcome of her husband's emergency surgery. She explained how her husband's heart surgery a month ago was followed yesterday by a massive stroke. They were working on him now, trying to save his life, and things didn't look good.

No sooner was I called to be registered for my angiogram than I got into a tiff with the supervising cardiologist. He wrote on his order "check renal artery." I insisted on knowing why they intended to examine the renal artery. Rather than simply saying that it was a common practice to check blood supply to the kidneys during angiograms, he replied by saying that I didn't have to have the test at all if I wished. I told him that I was just interested in what was happening to me.

Dressed in a gown, I was wheeled away. They shaved my groin area, cut open the artery, and installed an IV in my hand. Dosed with Valium, I was at first peaceful, but I became anxious as my wait dragged on for more than an hour. I was told they had an emergency ahead of me. First Lil's husband, now this—it must be rush hour on the Chicago thruway.

Finally, my appointed time came. They wheeled me into a relatively small room and had me scoot myself onto a narrow table. I lay on my back and looked at the machinery to my left and at the screen above. The doctor and his team were pleasant. We chatted, and I watched with amusement as the little creature wiggled its way up and around and darted back and forth inside my heart. I enjoyed myself, was proud of my cheery calm, even though I was never entirely unconscious of the fact that the innocent-seeming probing could, at any moment, incite a heart attack.

When they were done with me, I was wheeled back to the recovery room. A flat brick was used to close the wound in my groin area. I held the brick for the several hours I was kept in recovery. Later, confident that I had stabilized, they wheeled me up to a room, one of a dozen or so in the cardiac ward that formed a horseshoe around a large central nurses' desk. It held a bank of monitors that displayed the individual heart patterns of the patients on the ward. Alone in the room, my own heart monitor, to which I was tethered, constantly ticked away. It announced again and again and again: You are alive! You are alive! Yes, you are alive!

The cardiologist with whom I had had a tiff in the morning finally appeared late that afternoon. I was now to hear the news I had waited for. He was precise and brief. He told me that I had complete blockage of the left anterior descending coronary artery (LAD), which they could ideally bypass using the mammary artery, and 40 to 60 percent blockage in two other important left side arteries of the heart, which they would bypass with vein grafts from my legs.

He told me I was lucky. My heart was strong and undamaged. Nevertheless, I had significant blockage on the heart's dominant left side, although the blockage was partially mitigated by collateral vessels that provided alternative supplies of blood. To the question of a bypass, he replied that I could go either way. So I pressed, asking him which way he would go. He said he loved singles tennis, and to be able to play the game full-bore, he would have the bypass.

That answered it for me: I wouldn't. I preferred doubles

racquetball. I'd see what I could do with diet and exercise rather than permit such a massive intrusion of my body. I would, at least for the time being, bypass having a bypass.

I spent the evening resting in bed, only occasionally getting up to walk around the large horseshoe monitoring station at the center of the nearly empty ward. I could watch my own heartbeat as I moved. I could go only so far down the tangential halls without breaking contact with the station. On one trip, I encountered an older fellow patient accompanied by his wife. We talked with the immediate intimacy born of sharing a threatening condition. He was sixty-five. He had experienced a small heart attack. He was going to have a bypass and spoke about its promise. I did the best I could to explain why I had chosen to wait.

I didn't reflect on my condition that night. On my mind was only the wish to not have open-heart surgery and the doctor's assuring words that my condition didn't require it. In any case, even had I wanted to think about my heart, I wasn't equipped to do so. I knew only the most elemental information about the human heart: It is a pump at the center of a system of arteries and veins that gathers and disburses blood. It receives deoxygenated blood from the body and sends this blood to the lungs for oxygen. Then it redistributes the newly oxygenated blood back to the body. The body needs oxygen; oxygen is food for the cells.

Beyond that, the heart for me was a mix of metaphors and myths. It might as well have been the whole continent of Africa. With no interest in anatomy and even less in engineering, I appreciated neither the heart's sensitivity nor its endurance as a mechanism. While the normal human heart rate is seventy-two beats per minute (in contrast to Beluga whales, which have a heart rate of fifteen beats per minute, and shrews, the smallest of mammals, which have a heart rate of a thousand beats per minute), the human heart can beat less than fifty beats per minute and more than two hundred, in addition to changing its volume to meet the body's needs. Supplied with an automatic sensor, the heart continually responds to the slightest movements of body and mind over a lifetime. At sixty beats per minute, it supplies five quarts of blood to the body in one minute. At the same rate, it supplies 1,800 gallons a day, 657,000 gallons a year, and 46,000,000 gallons in a seventy-year lifetime.

Only later, after I read books and articles, did I learn that the average human heart is about the size of two human fists and weighs about three-fourths of a pound (which is considerably less than the estimated thousand-pound heart of a large great blue whale). I would have to examine models of the heart to grasp the different functions of the two sides and their two chambers (the right receives the returning blood and pumps it to the lungs, while the left sends the oxygenated blood to the body). At the time, I had no idea how the relaxing (diastole) of the heart allows blood returning from the body to flow into the upper right chamber, the atrium, and down into the lower right chamber, the ventricle. At the same time it allows blood returning from the lungs to flow into the upper left atrium and then down into the lower left ventricle. Alternately, the constriction (systole) of the heart ejects blood from the lower right ventricle to the lungs and, at the same time, the lower left ventricle to the body. I was unaware that electrical impulses cause the bellows-like pumping movement of the heart and that the valves at the chambers' entrances and exits assure the advance of the blood in a single direction.

I knew as much about my heart as I knew about the pumps under the hood of my car, which was next to nothing. I did know atherosclerotic heart disease was common in epidemic proportions in contemporary history, causing a good portion of the 500,000 deaths by heart disease that occur in this country each year. I realized that it was a newer explanation for those who once died merely of heart failure, congestive heart failure, or even the once popularly diagnosed acute indigestion. I knew, thanks to Kacz's explanations, that its basic cause is the buildup of materials in the coronary arteries. At some point these materials (which accumulate as part of the aging process) stop the coronary arteries from furnishing oxygen to the heart. Like any other muscle denied oxygen, the heart goes into a spasm, leaving it unable to supply blood to itself and the body. On this basis, I understood that a heart attack involves the death of part, or the whole, of the heart.

My wife had alerted me to how certain kinds of fats cause cholesterol, surely the source of heart blockage and the most notorious and best known culprit of heart attacks. I also had been told that smoking, which I had continued for about twenty-five years, from age twelve to age thirty-seven, and intuitively held responsible for my condition, caused lesions to which cholesterol and plaque stick, forming arterial blockage. Even though Cathy and my doctors helped me grasp the relationship of atherosclerosis (which causes one's arteries to be inelastic) and high blood pressure (toward which I had a tendency), I had no idea how much blockage one could have before having a heart attack became a virtual certainty, and I had no feel for calculating how collateral circulation might be developed to deliver an alternative supply of blood to the heart. I didn't doubt that I was truly in danger, although I suspected that a heart attack could be statistically anticipated but never precisely predicted.

But that night I did not suffer my ignorance or suspicions, nor was I bothered by the fact that my beating heart was tethered to a distant monitor. I fell asleep easily, and I slept well and long.

I woke the next day and was ready to go home. I had suffered only the mildest discomforts—the worst of which was having to lie still for several hours with a brick on the wound in the groin area where the probe had entered my body. Discharged as scheduled the next morning, I left for home with my sister-in-law. I felt like Jonah spewed up on the beach. I had been in the belly of the beast, the hospital, and escaped it. It had not killed me; it had not kept me, or even ordered me to come back.

Even though so little had happened and I was only slightly scarred, I nevertheless left the hospital a different person from the one who went in. My character remained the same. My projects were unaltered. My family and social relationships were not transformed. Yet I had been marked in a special way. Heart disease would stalk me hereafter — and in all likelihood, would get me in the end.

My autonomy had been violated. My heart had been entered. I would carry with me both in my mind and folded in my wallet a diagram of my blocked heart. On the front, it indicated which arteries were blocked; on the back it listed the doctors' findings. In one of my front pockets, I carried a small brown bottle of nitroglycerin pills. I stationed duplicates of the little bottle in the drawer of my nightstand, on my desk at work, and in my gym locker. They kept falling out of my pockets, cropping up on the dresser, collecting at the bottom of my golf bags. They were a constant reminder that I was marked out.

As never before, not even when as a boy I strove to perfect my golf swing to become a professional, I was joined to an ongoing conversation with my body. Obsessively, I listened inwardly. I scrutinized the subtlest sensations for the first indications of serious symptoms. Consciousness became a nervous threshold across which my body's pulsations constantly crossed. When I ran or walked quickly, I noted my breathing, which measured how my heart was performing. Almost compulsively, I would reach for my wrist and take my pulse. I especially did this in church. The pulse in my wrist was an outpost of my heart, but even when my pulse was strong and regular, the powerful throbbing sound no longer assured me of my vitality.

Weighing myself regularly was another part of my conversation with my body. I was intense and precise about it. I took my weight, which had dropped since my diagnosis, as a measure of my fat and, thus, as the measure of the wellness of my heart. I also took it as a measure of how sincere I was about taking care of myself and preventing a bypass.

All this placed me — as I knew full well — on the doorstep of hypochondria. I feared I would transform myself into one of those people who measure the days by symptoms and imagined diseases. But this fear didn't keep me from my constant self-monitoring. I asked my wife to take my blood pressure two or three times a day. Out on my regular biking trips, I frequently sneaked to the nearby drugstore and used its blood pressure machine, as if I were committing a secret sin, hoping its numbers would supply me the healing information my anxiety both sought and denied me. However, I was forever disappointed. My varying blood pressure only produced a bewildering array of numbers and additional anxiety. I simply couldn't pin down how I was doing.

Like the contemporary infected person, be it an HIV/AIDS victim or a cancer patient, I was preoccupied with invisible things. I knew that inside of me, at some microscopic level, minute particles were accumulating in me like fine silt. They were depositing themselves in layers of deadly blockage. My own coursing blood was delivering minute bits to deadly dams that over time would close my arteries. I sensed that at work within me were natural processes — so similar to those that form rocks, block rivers, and corrode pipes — that over time age and kill humans.

Each blood test turned the hour glass of time for me. It

measured whether the good cholesterol (the cleansing high-density, or HDL) or the bad cholesterol (the low-density sticking, or LDL) was increasing and whether or not the blockage was building. I tried to read my need for a bypass and the length of my life by the numbers I received from each lab test. While I knew that these numbers were only photographs of my blood at any one moment, my anxiety insisted that they offer more certain and fixed indications.

I thought of death more than ever. From childhood on I had thought of death. From the age of seven, possibly younger, I sensed that at some moment in time I would no longer be. I was preoccupied with death in my late teens and twenties and so frequently wrote on death in my thirties and forties. Now I had reason to think even more about what I could know so little.

⌒—⧸⧸—⌒

A question arose almost immediately after my discharge from the hospital. Should I take a planned trip to Uruguay to visit my oldest daughter, Felice? The cardiologist saw no reason why I couldn't. So off I went, preoccupied with my diet, pulse, breathing, and heart.

The trip started from Minneapolis. I had a long stopover in Miami, where I spent an afternoon walking the Cuban neighborhood of Calle Ocho, intensely thinking about my heart, reading Spanish signs, eating a meal of fish without butter, and wondering where in Miami Beach my father, mother, and I had stayed when I was a boy forty years before. Later, from the plane, I watched the great muddy river, the Amazon, and thought of the blood flowing through me.

My daughter and I spent our first full day in Buenos Aires going from police station to police station looking for her passport, which had been lifted by a pickpocket at our first supper together. With a sour taste in our mouths, we left Buenos Aires for Montevideo, where I stayed near the great bay formed by the Rio de la Plata as it emptied into the sea. Each day after spending time with my daughter and visiting friends, art museums, and vegetarian restaurants, I would eat my oat bran, walk briskly along the beach walkway filled with joggers and dogs, and then meditate and relax. I continued to monitor my heart and listen to my body. I frequently weighed myself on scales in the streets and wished I could lose weight faster. I wanted to go from 216 pounds to 175 as quickly as possible. As I walked ever greater lengths at nearby beaches and when we later traveled in southern Brazil, I steadily regained confidence in my body. I remembered how, when I caddied as a boy, I could walk and run as far as I wanted to go.

I cleared a great hurdle in making the trip to see my daughter: My heart condition had not tethered me to home. I could live beyond my fears.

This did not mean that I felt free to do anything I wanted. There was a kind of ascetic discipline to my life now. I had to watch what and how much I ate and drank. I had to stick to an exercise regimen. I slit my gargantuan throat with my own hand to live longer. I ate less and better. Thanks to my wife, I ate more greens, learned to cook with a wok, and, while never embracing the vegetarian ideal, I used vegetarian recipes and shared, no doubt for the wrong reasons, an aversion to eating too much meat. I did what the good dieter should do, as best my wife, the nurse and nutritionist, could explain it to me. My weight dropped to 185, where I encountered a wall.

I exercised regularly. I read books on exercise, cholesterol, and aerobics, and even books about how longtime cardiac patients had turned into marathon runners. I wanted to believe that I could reverse my heart damage. As I first learned to jog, each session seemed perilous as I inched my heart rate up into the 120s and held it there for ten, then fifteen, then twenty, and finally thirty, forty, and, on occasion, even fifty minutes. Initially, I was giddy and ecstatic with my progress. It was as if I were traveling over the abyss to new heights.

I learned to jog in tune with my breathing. I focused on distant sights, and often slowly prayed the Our Father as I ran. I made each part of the prayer a separate evocation and meditation. Between "Our Father" and "Who Art in Heaven," I ran hundreds of yards. When I ran, I felt awake, alive, often with God.

It was as if I ran with, against, and beyond death. I was doing what I should have learned to do long before this heart condition. I let things come as they would. Alone with myself, I ran on God's grace.

Exercise (thirty or forty minutes of it every day or every other day) became a great delight. I added a rowing machine to the exercise bike in my basement. I took my ice skates out of the closet and soon, at rinks at home and far away, I was again one of the better skaters on the ice. I took delight in the sense of speed and gliding. I took my swimming suit and jump rope on trips. I rode my racing bike ten, twenty, and thirty miles at a crack in the city and out into the surrounding countryside. I played doubles racquetball. I took three or four three-mile walks a week and played golf, which I, an old caddie, contend can only be played properly by walking. Exercise was my pleasure, my ascesis, and my ecstasy.

I also fooled with medicine and vitamins. I introduced massive doses (2,000 to 2,500 milligrams) of niacin into my diet, following the recommendation of one of the books I read. I saw my total cholesterol (LDLs) fall as low as 160 or so and my good, protective cholesterol (HDLs) rise to 50, which was a vast improvement over the 240-over-29 at the time of my diagnosis.

I also got my temper under better control. This meant recognizing how often and how quickly I got angry. I noted how I brought a lot of passion to confronting insoluble situations and unchangeable personalities. I tried to escape those countless occasions for anger abundantly furnished at home and at work. I purposely withheld attributing any significance to many of the affairs of everyday life. I resisted, as best I could, having an opinion on everything. I often succeeded in ducking people and situations I never would have avoided in the past. Indifference and silence began to serve me well. I consistently refused requests to go to political and academic meetings, and felt good about it. An ideal meeting in town or school, I joked, was one that occurred at the same time as another, so I could miss not just one but both. I became suspicious of actions that depended on collaboration with others who, in the majority, I judged to be doing as little as possible. I became more dubious of administrative promises, which were usually based on present needs, scanty visions, and fickle loyalties. I restricted myself to doing things I could control and that had realizable ends. All this had the consequence of directing more and more of my energies to writing projects, which at least ended in the tangible results of books.

I paid particular attention to the process of how anger rose up in me. I realized that I was at my worst on the days I was coming down with a cold. Then my irritability was greatest and the clarity of my mind weakest. Unfortunately, I usually discovered the onset of a cold after being exceptionally angry about a small thing. I did find morning exercise helpful in tapping my piss and vinegar before I went to work at Southwest State University, a small rural college on the Minnesota prairie. The school is usually astir with anxiety and often spinning with accusation. This was primarily due to constant administrative turnover, intermittent budgetary shortfalls, and episodes of faculty rivalry and resentment, which dashed any hope for the quiet and calm of the examined life. If I did get angry at work, I would go jump rope or jog in the gym. I realized that the college, in which I had sunk almost twenty-five years of my life and which provided me a decent salary, a few good friends, and some good students, was not in business to make me happy. It could even play a role in killing me off if I took it too seriously. So it was, I concluded, and it never would be different.

Though a long way from mastering the art of quietness, I had achieved a certain calm. I found solace in reading St. Paul's message that God's salvation comes from Christ rather than from me, and that it includes people of hot tempers and nervous energy as much as those of Buddha-like calm. Increasingly freed from obsession with health and heart, I took my pulse and blood pressure less and less often.

In the meantime, while a rehabilitation cardiologist reconfirmed my condition with a radioactive treadmill test and an ecocardiagram (which in retrospect seemed more costly than instructive), Kacz and I worked out a simple plan. It pleased my sense of reason: We would continue to monitor my blood with quarterly tests and checkups and annual stress tests. Our goal would be for me to last as long as I could without a bypass. If I lasted ten years, I would be sixty. With the average bypass lasting fifteen years, I might make it beyond what seemed to me the wonderfully biblical age of seventy.

At one point, Kacz optimistically postulated that by the time I needed a bypass, surgeons would be using far less intrusive laser surgery. After a year or so of talking about it, I went to the University of Minnesota medical library and read about laser surgery. From my reading I deduced that the successful use of laser surgery, especially with patients with an occluded main artery like mine, lay in the future. Meanwhile, I felt on the right track: Run, test, pray, hope, and see what happens.

⟨⟨⟨

In December 1993, a little more than five years after my first diagnosis, I was again at the Minneapolis Heart Institute at Abbott Northwestern for a stress test with my cardiologist, Doctor James Daniels. If it came out like the recent one I had

had in Marshall, I would take the angiogram he had already scheduled for the following day. I remembered having spoken of the possibility of a second angiogram five years before. I was told that wasn't in the protocol. Yet, there I was, being asked to drive to Chicago again.

I assumed that since he had ordered the angiogram in advance, the stress test would, in all likelihood, call for a look inside. Before the results of the test in Marshall, I had found myself faltering when I jogged, feeling more listless, and once even having trouble walking on a hot, humid night. I interpreted this to mean that my heart wasn't getting as much oxygen as it should.

I had prepared for the test at Abbott Northwestern like a fighter training for a prize fight. I felt like a person being summoned to the highest court of stewardship to be asked how well I had taken care of my closest friend, my body. Nevertheless, as determined as I was to take that test, when I got out of bed that morning, I didn't believe I could manage it. I literally hobbled about because of what I thought was gout, rheumatism, or a bruise on my right big toe joint. My toe had given me trouble for a whole week before, and now, on the eve of the test, it had flared up so badly that even a sheet resting upon it caused me pain. Nevertheless, as the morning wore on and it loosened up, and thanks to my cardiologist's encouragement, I managed to take the test. After what for me was a near effortless, and I thought stellar, nine-minute performance on the treadmill, he took me off. He didn't like what he saw. He suspected increased blockage.

I was additionally humiliated. Unexplainably, my total cholesterol test returned with a stunning 271. I hoped that the protective HDL at 59 helped my body more than my pride. My cholesterol hadn't been that high in five years. I felt like a failure.

In the skillful hands of the taciturn woman cardiologist who carried it out, the angiogram caused me no discomfort. However, it confirmed what my doctors suspected: more blockage. My left anterior descending artery was still entirely occluded; the two other blocked arteries on the left side had gone from 40 to 80 percent and from 60 to 90 percent.

Doctor Daniels's recommendation was unequivocally for a bypass. I translated his sparse words and even sparser show of emotions, whose pilot light seemed a gentle melancholy, into the risk numbers he gave me for a bypass. They were reprinted on a card I was handed: a 3 percent risk of dying, 12 percent chance of a stroke, 15 percent chance for heart muscle damage, 15 percent chance for early closure of the bypass graft. In my case, he elaborated in response to my questions, given my age, chances of dying were roughly 2 percent, and this 2 percent included those 12 percent who would have a stroke during or as a consequence of the operation. The vast majority of incidences of heart muscle damage were insignificant.

They would use a large vein from my leg to bypass two partially occluded arteries. The left mammary artery graft that they would use for bypassing my occluded artery, he assured me, was a highly desirable bypass. While once considered a surgically more difficult operation, the mammary artery had a larger diameter than the vein to be harvested from my leg, which meant more blood for my heart and greater likelihood that the bypass would stay open longer. I had fully entered the web of their techniques and explanations.

And if I didn't get the bypass? I queried. Each year there would be a 10 percent chance that I would have a heart attack. Furthermore, there was a good chance that it would be severe. As Doctor Odland had surmised five years before, he believed there was also a good chance the attack might come without warning, which played against the odds that I would make it to the hospital (which I later read assures a patient a 90 percent survival rate) or that I would make it to the hospital quickly, where new medicines can in many cases mitigate the damage caused by a heart attack.

So, I had to judge incalculable probabilities and eventualities. They couldn't be tallied with certainty. Like a stiff new pair of shoes, they could only be gotten used to. I was thrown into a numbers game with mortal consequences, feeling that I didn't quite know all the numbers on the dice or the odds. In the end, as I knew from the start, I understood full well that my calculations depended on instinct and judgment. I would think one thing with one part of my mind, only to conclude something else with another. I also grasped trouble on two sides: I had to refuse collapsing into the arms of their authority, on the one hand, yet I didn't want to flinch before the operation because of fear of death on the other. I was mildly amused that such deadly business should come in such a sophisticated form.

At the same time, I sensed death looming ahead, lurking in my arteries. I told the doctor I would go home and think it over.

The absence of pain made my considerations difficult. As is often true for those with heart trouble, pain had not yet stepped on my chest or taken me by the throat and thrown me down. I had not even experienced angina. I was free of symptoms. Aside from a little burping now and then and a few incidences of shortness of breath, I was still able to outskate, outgolf, and outbike most people. Yet I at fifty-five had to consider an operation that included the risk of death and stroke.

For a few days I played with the odds like a riverboat gambler, as if somehow the odds could be used to weigh a life against death. At worst, the odds, as I figured them, were about 33 to 1 that I would die or suffer a serious stroke during the operation. (I assumed that some of those who died of the bypass died of strokes, and I believed my age and condition gave me an edge.) These were not bad odds. If I were drawing from a full deck of cards, the odds were two to three times better than drawing an ace, which was one out of thirteen. They were roughly equal to the odds of throwing snake eyes or boxcars, which is one out of thirty-six. As boy I had spent enough time on my knees, alongside the old ice box amid uncles who were rolling craps, to know that these were damn good odds. But my uncles only lost a few bucks when the wrong sides of their dice came up.

I was trying to weigh what could not be weighed. Instead of numbers, I thought that ahead of me lay a narrow but deep ditch that I had to leap. Chances of not making it were slight. But the ditch was as deep as death itself. Of course, life, I thought, often turns on the unexpected. There is always a mistake, an overlooked detail, a surprising occurrence resulting in an unforeseen tragedy. The black queen turns up at odd times.

I frequently left the realm of probabilities, hypotheses, and statistics for that of metaphors. How else, except with metaphors, could I weigh this real life against that imagined death? My mother had told me repeatedly throughout my childhood, even after I had done something wrong, Deep down, you've a good heart. As much as anything, this compliment gave me a moral spine. I prided myself on having a good heart.

After a lifetime of treating my heart as my moral center, I couldn't simply let it be reduced to a mere object of medical practice. A heart, at least as poets would have it, is more than what seventeenth-century English scientist William Harvey described as a small muscular pump. Heir, as I was, of such powerful and diverse legions of metaphors associated with the word *heart,* how could I think of my heart coldly, as the children of Harvey do? In this operation they would stop my heart (Isn't that death?), pack it in ice (Aren't hearts meant to be warm?), fill it with salts, and turn instruments, knives, and needles upon the organ that harbors my passions and enthusiasms. They were going to ply their technology on the single heart upon whose pulsing beat my life has ever depended.

They would enter into me. They would saw my breast bone in two, cleave and pry my chest wide open, and begin the terribly precise and bloody practice of their craft.

Yet, they promised what I wanted: a longer and fuller earthly life. I was willing to put on their silly gown, lie unconscious and supine upon their table, and pay the price of physical discomfort and metaphorical dissonance they would cause with their surgery on my heart.

After all, to make a confession I had just learned to make: I am a modern. Like everyone else, I want less pain and more pleasure. I certainly was not going to stand on principle and refuse the surgery that promised me a long life just because surgeons have a long history of robbing graves, exploiting the dead in poor houses, or developing the field of heart surgery at the expense of stray dogs and occasional baboons.

Juggling statistics wasn't going to determine what I should do. They might have put an end to much of my deliberations if the odds were 1,000 to 1 against anything going wrong, but this wasn't the case. The simplest resolution would have been to surrender my will to the experts' knowledge. But that didn't fit my style. And it didn't square with my self-image as a critical thinking college professor. Thinking and talking about things was my normal, if clumsy and pretentious, way to substantiate my earnestness.

I traversed layers and layers of superstitions as I thought about my condition. I have always been filled with superstitions and suspected I would never get beyond them. My superstitions were not about the names of doctors, nor did I have holy medals, lucky rings, or required rituals. Rather, I took certain days of the week to be more auspicious than others. (I have always preferred Wednesday over Tuesday or

Thursday.) I have certain prayers that must be said, and I feel more secure if I have certain things in my pocket (like a small pocketknife or a notebook to record my thoughts).

Irrational ideas about numbers, particularly about my age, assembled themselves and wandered my mind like half-drunk men. Since childhood, I had feared bad things from even numbers, especially four and eight, and expected good things from odd numbers, especially three and seven. Under even numbers, I believed I would harvest the bad things of life: misfortune, disease, and death. This fantasizing over numbers had persisted throughout my life, even though it contradicted the fact that I was blessedly born in the eighth month of 1938 and in the same month in 1966 I blessedly married my wife.

Even though I never transferred my belief in numbers to astrology, my defiant mind tenaciously clung to the idea that fifty-five—a double five—was an auspicious age for a bypass. Five was an odd number; it was about life, not death, as the prefatory quotation by Scot Morris to my friend Philip Dacey's book, *Fives*, confirms:

> In biology the number five crops up more than its share of times. Practically all land vertebrates have five fingers and five toes. . . . Many marine animals, including sea urchins, sand dollars, and sea cucumbers, have five-fold symmetry. Most modern starfish have five arms. . . . Most flowers have five petals, and even those that have many more, such as the daisy, have an underlying five-fold symmetry. Many fruits show the quintessence of their ancestry: Cut an apple, a pear, or a banana crosswise and you'll see the seeds are arranged in a five-pointed star.

However fine the number five is, I wanted to shout out, it is all right for a starfish to be cut in half in order to be regenerated, but why should I, a human being, have to be cut in half, or nearly in half, so that I would have a long life? Why should a surgeon have to break my chest bone, which would be the first bone ever broken in my body, so that my heart would throb and thump with rushing blood and I would be free, at least for a while, of the heart disease that had stalked my consciousness for the past five years? I remembered how I had reacted to the first bypass I saw on television: The doctors sawed and pried open a man's chest. They exposed the patient's raw, beating heart. Once it no longer moved, they meticulously worked with their knives and needles upon it. I had said to myself, better dead than that.

I was also not free of what others consider more profound superstitions. I believed that somehow God, in spite of the infinity of human and animal voices, hears individual prayers. He intervenes in and even supersedes the laws of nature for the sake of a single person. He can and does intercede in the infinity of things, from the greatest to the smallest, to perform miracles. I also believed that God, on occasion, might defy the opinions of scientists and doctors and allow a lame person to walk again. However, I balked at the notion that God would defy nature to the point of allowing an armless and legless person to grow new limbs.

An even greater superstition was that I, an only child and son, was special. I was hypnotized to this faith by my very name, Amato, which means in Italian, the beloved. In my whole life, I had never experienced the idea that no one cared about me. I always felt I had an interested audience in family, friends, and God himself. Indeed, my sense of self-importance was so immense, that even if I concluded that not a single person cared what happened to me, I still would have believed myself to be an object of importance. Even though I assented to fate, I never felt abandoned to indifferent forces. My diagnosis did not lead me to believe that my fate turned simply on debris in my coronary arteries and merely on the skill of a surgeon's hands.

Other beliefs, like the poles of a teepee, formed my tent under the skies. I believed that if I made it off the operating table, I would recover. Despite my heart troubles, I have always assumed that I have been blessed by a healthy body that is capable of rejuvenation. I also assumed that my family was meant to live to old age, partly because I believed that my grandfather, who died of appendicitis when he was only thirty-three, had ransomed the rest of us from early deaths.

At the same time, since I had first seriously begun reading books, I had expected an early death. I interpreted the soft tinge of melancholy that I saw in my own eye as a signal of a premature rendezvous with death. As much as I would claim that I didn't lend any credence to palmistry, I continually glanced at the life line that curved from the outer edge of my right palm to the wrist. I took its early branching as a signal of life-threatening crises in middle life and frequently scanned its path for confirmation that I had indeed made it through that first branching.

This romantic tendency to expect an early death in an age of increasing longevity was never accompanied by any distinct premonition of how and where I would die. And I had no sense whatsoever whether my death would fulfill my life or prove a nasty irony. From time to time, I even thought that preoccupying myself with my mortality (which could take every form my imagination could impress on it) was simply a waste of time.

Nevertheless, thinking about death was something I had done since my early youth. It was a lens through which I looked at life. It was a kind of poetry for me. It made life less certain, less secure, hence more dramatic and urgent. It joined me to that odd company of medieval monks who studied with skulls on their desks; Renaissance poets, who reminded us how quickly life passes into death; and skaters, who, moving on cutting blades, listen for the sound of cracking ice as they move over dark water.

Keeper of the Graves

Ten days before my surgery was scheduled, I went on a trip to Detroit I had planned earlier to visit my father's and grandparents' graves. I spent three days there making provisional farewells to them and the world I knew as a boy.

When my father died five years earlier, I became the family keeper of the graves. My mother, who came to Minnesota to live with us shortly after his death, was too broken in spirit to ever return to Detroit. So I was obligated to make an annual visit to the resting places of the dead. The older I grew, the more the dead took a hold of me. I considered my heart a temple in which they resided, and I acknowledged the strong but undefined duty to complete their lives with mine.

Visiting the dead on the eve of my bypass made me edgy. I was uncertain whether I would merely once again be paying my respects or announcing my imminent reunion with them. I felt that I might soon be as alive as they were alive or as dead as they were dead. I knew that when I was no longer around to remember them, they would be forgotten, and that I was on the verge of slipping into the same abyss.

Before going to Mount Olivet Cemetery, where my family was buried, I drove with a friend named Ted Radzilowski to the east side of Detroit. We headed for the Walter Reuther AUW-CIO retirement high-rise on the Detroit River where former ethnic labor organizer Stanley Nowak and his wife, Margaret, lived. Ted had written a preface to Stanley's autobiography. Stanley, dying of cancer, wanted to see Ted one last time and give him the last batch of books from his library.

The trip through the east side was for me a trip into my past. My mother's family arrived on the east side of Detroit from the Fox River Valley area of Wisconsin in the 1920s. Her restless mother, Frances, moved the family from house to house (sometimes as often as twice a year) on the east side of Detroit and, now and then, out to the surrounding lakes and up north to the woods. In her youth my mother attended a dozen Detroit schools because of her mother's inability to stay in one place. I remember from my own youth another dozen east side houses my grandmother lived in. There were so many that when we drove to visit her we frequently found ourselves heading for the wrong house. She never found stability in life, and I knew her flux in some measure now to mortally be mine.

My dad's family also lived on Detroit's east side, where they arrived from Pennsylvania coal fields just before the First World War. At first they lived downtown, as that generation of Italian immigrants did. Then they bought a house three miles east of downtown, in the Charlevoix and St. Jean area. For his whole working life of more than fifty years my dad rode buses across the east side of Detroit to his work downtown, first from his family home and then from his own homes, one at Six Mile and Harper and the other at Eight Mile and Gratiot.

As a boy I rode the same bus lines. I also remember the Jefferson Avenue electric streetcar line. As the cars gently accelerated, swaying as they went, I watched the unused leather straps swing in unison high above the wicker benches. I knew the east side well. I had pondered its gigantic factories surrounded by fields of tanks, trucks, and jeeps, shopped many of its stores, played ball on many of its fields, and rode my bike down and across many of its side streets.

The Nowaks, who lived just off Jefferson, belonged to the world of 1930s unionism to which my father and mother also belonged. As Ted Radzilowski wrote in his preface to Stanley's autobiography, they numbered among the leaders who helped fashion a unionized working class out of Detroit's ethnic communities, especially the Poles.

Hardly had we entered their small ninth-floor apartment than Stanley, in his early nineties, got down to the business of beginning what seemed to me his often repeated recollections. With occasional help from Margaret, he told us about how he made his entrance into the world of radical labor politics. His debut turned out to be nothing other than the Palmer Raids of 1919. Inspired by postwar communist hysteria, the raids targeted foreigners and social radicals throughout the nation. A fourteen-year-old journalist for a Chicago Polish-American paper, Stanley was asked to go to the police station to serve as a translator for the Poles who had been rounded up. This experience defined his basic sympathies and was the basis of a commitment that led him to the center of radical labor organizing in Detroit during the Depression.

Stanley's speech confidently flowed like the great river below his apartment. He made the best of his last chance to provide Ted with his version of history. I had no room in myself for his remembrance. Measured against my death, his stories and ideas, which went hand and hand, seemed remote, devoid of the transcendence I sought.

I slipped out onto his apartment balcony. I stood in a pale but warming early morning December light. Below, the mighty Detroit River rushed by in rising swells. Once, when I was a boy, just downriver from Stanley and Margaret's apartment, at the foot of the pilings of the Belle Isle Bridge, my father and I saw a super hydroplane take flight because of those swells. It flipped over and upside down and ploughed the water until it stopped. The driver was killed. Later, as part of the crowd that lined the shore, we solemnly watched the ripped and broken hydroplane towed back to dock, its strutting showing through its torn hull. I felt that I was approaching the swells of a dangerous course.

As a boy, in the days preceding the transfer of the world championship of unlimited hydroplanes to Seattle, I loved to hear those wonderful machines winding themselves up on the river. Their deep roar resonated up and down the whole east side. They were like giant animals straining on their leashes. With large Allison and Rolls Royce motors, these unlimited hydroplanes, with names like *Tempo I, Miss Canada,* and *Skip-Along,* roared and hummed, and squealed when they took flight from the water.

I could clearly see Belle Isle, Detroit's pearl of an island, from Stanley and Margaret's apartment. On that island, generations of Detroit eastsiders pursued their pleasures. We drove our cars to the island to kill time, date, or, to use a phrase from my youth, "watch the submarine races." On the island we picnicked, canoed, swam, visited the small zoo, watched miniature boat races, went to the annual aquarama, rode bikes and horses, skated the canals in winter, and watched the passing giant freighters and ore ships that connected us to Lake Superior in one direction and the Atlantic Ocean in the other. Once, near the end of the Second World War, the U.S. Army even staged a mock beach landing on the island for the public, with landing vehicles and hundreds of soldiers.

My parents' generation went to the island for wedding pictures, a favorite spot being Scott Fountain. My mother told me stories about Belle Isle, how she and her classmates collected money to purchase an elephant for the zoo, and how she won a grade school hurdles race there. She also told me how my dad, no athlete, played tennis on the island, and how her favorite aunt, Aunt May—a nurse and a woman well ahead of her time—threw her golf clubs in one of the island's canals when one of her dubbed shots went into the water. I have two photographs of my mother as a young woman on Belle Isle. Slender, dressed in white, she and her friends are playing croquet. In another picture, she sits romantically in a large and branching tree like a flower.

When I stepped back inside the apartment, Stanley and Margaret were getting out the last boxes of books Ted was to take. Unlike earlier books they had given him, which represented a life of reading in politics, social and labor history, and science, these were the leftovers: a jumble of mediocre and didactic texts. The worst had been saved for last.

As I helped load the boxes into a grocery cart to haul them down to the lobby, where a handful of old retired union workers were congregated, I thought how little a lifelong collection of books means once it leaves its original owner's hands. I remembered how little my forty-seven-year-old colleague and friend Maynard Brass's books meant to the world. We couldn't even find a library to take them. I knew that one day my books would be as senselessly disbursed as those of Maynard and Stanley.

Ted and the Nowaks' goodbyes were brief. Stanley had asked Ted to say his eulogy at the commemorative service. Stanley, socialist intellectual, had delivered himself into the hands of Ted, a Catholic, but also, perhaps savingly, a unionist and fellow Pole, and surely Stanley's best hope of being remembered.

As we left the grounds of the Walter Reuther housing project, I felt relieved. We were leaving behind the burden of trying to be alive to what was dying. We were driving away from Stanley's and his generation's claim on our memory. We were light, fragile vehicles trying to escape the gravity of their past.

Less than a mile down Jefferson Avenue, we passed what was once the great pride of Detroit: the city waterworks. In its heyday, Detroit pumped water in greater quantities than did most other industrial cities. With its water and numerous tree-lined streets, Detroit was a model of cleanliness and shade. My parents, like most of their generation, took great pride in the city's water system, as well as its green lawns, trees, and parks. And they took pride in the city's teams (especially the Tigers), its athletes (Joe Lewis, most notably), and its industrial production, which made it the carmaker of the world and "the arsenal of democracy." I can remember how, with each census, they cheered their town's growth—for a time it was the fourth-largest city in the nation. They believed they were the makers of a marvelous metropolis. They cherished their identity with the city more than that with the nation. Detroit's water seemed to make them immortal.

The east side we now passed through was not the one of my parents' pride. On the way to the cemetery, we saw neighborhood after neighborhood of empty stores and abandoned houses. There were even boarded-up storefront churches. Whole blocks, where houses once stood, were fields of uncut weeds. There were miles of dilapidated homes on whose driveways stood cars stranded on blocks. One school we passed had a lawn ill-kept, more of weeds than grass, on which stood a few dying crab apple trees.

We entered the grounds of Mount Olivet Cemetery, where society held back the surrounding chaos of the east side. Here in the garden of the dead, the lawn was watered and mowed, the trees flourished, and nothing was broken or littered. Even though I would be buried in Minnesota if anything were to happen, I felt I belonged to this cemetery, which held so much of my family and my early memories of death and burial.

In the vast cemetery among curving roads, I found my father's graveside with little effort. I made use of the large monument across the lane from him. The name on it was, phonetically, "Dee Dee." My mother teased that Dee Dee was a former bubble dancer who paid my father nightly visits.

On his stone, it said only: "Beloved Husband and Father 1912-1989." No moral or narrative of his life was offered. It didn't say, as it should have, that he was a man who gave his life for work and family. He was the son of impoverished Sicilian immigrants, and his father died when he was three years old. When his stepfather was put in prison, he took full responsibility for the family. After graduating from high school at sixteen, he went to work for Western Union, where he stayed for the next forty-three years. He held many important positions in the company and every post in Western Union's union before joining management. In all that time, he missed only two days of work.

As I gazed at my father's headstone, the notion came to me that he had died first to lead the way through death for the rest of us. I remembered once when he, my mother, and I were at the edge of a large woods. A large wolf, or wolf-like dog, approached us. My father picked up a great stick to fight the dog and jammed us into an outdoor toilet. My mother and I stayed there in the dark until the dog went away, and my father called us out. Would he protect me during my bypass, I found myself asking.

Or perhaps he died first because he was tired. He had worked the hardest and worried the most. He took care of his mother and raised his own sister and three stepsisters before he started his own family. Perhaps life had squeezed the juice out of him. He certainly didn't have the zip my mother had—but few did, especially when she was in one of her high moods. Perhaps he went first because God deemed him the most ready to enter heaven. My father always met his obligations and consistently did what he thought was right. He never held grudges, and he forgave people easily. I was not his equal in equanimity, and it was too late, whatever the outcome of the bypass, for me—feisty, proud, and itchy—to match his character.

Even though little grass had grown up over his headstone, I still felt he had been left alone too long. He had died of a massive heart attack at age seventy-seven five years earlier. It had been two years since I had visited his graveside. I felt I had ignored him. In fact, I had never paid sufficient attention to him. As when he was alive, my mom gripped the limelight with her volatile personality and inconsistent health. Her mercurial personality often left my family with little energy to think about him or anything else.

As fathers and sons often do, my father and I had grown closer over the years. Our talk covered a range of things—

some sports, a little investing, and a fair amount of politics. In contrast to my mom, he rarely talked about his past. He made no effort to remember it or awaken feelings about it. He would complain about the Republicans, interest rates, or contemporary politics. Occasionally, in the last ten or so years, he would also complain about my mother. She would either be high — on "a talking jag" — or low. When I suggested the possibility of treatment, he argued that nothing could be done. He believed that her pride prohibited treatment, and he was probably right. Anyhow, he himself lent only grudging respect to medicine, and he had no place in his mind for psychology.

In his middle seventies, his self-prognosis was for a life to eighty. He almost always second-guessed his doctors. He freely drew his own conclusions from their opinions. He did concede that he had adult diabetes, and he made an effort to exercise, but he was too weak to do much. It was painful for me to see his legs weaken in his last years. He struggled to turn the pedals of my exercise bike. These legs, which had never failed him, now could not carry him a block to the corner store. My mother told me that the doctors had told her that he had the body of a very old man. This time her report may have been right. At such times I feared I was made of him rather than her. She would survive a bypass better.

The last time I saw him alive he told me about a serious bout of dizziness he had recently suffered. Just as he had finished shining his car, he had had to sit down for twenty minutes. During that last visit he explained his assets and showed me where he kept his papers and security box keys. He didn't dally. He didn't repeat himself. That was as close as we came to discussing what he may have sensed was his pending death.

It was understood that if anything happened to him, I would take over. Although my mother was marvelous at saving money, she had no understanding of banking and interest. He knew he had done his duty of providing for her welfare. He had formed a small estate that, coupled with her modest social security check, would keep her well. He had secured his family—first his mother and sisters, then his wife and son. My dad had earned his rest.

A rotund, good looking man, with a generous smile, my father was not particularly colorful. He was like the children of many immigrant families, especially those missing a parent: He was smart, responsible, and knew how to work. He was a man of duty. He didn't fight in the war as my uncles had. He didn't play sports—hardly skated, quit playing tennis in his early twenties, couldn't be coaxed to learn to golf or bowl, and really couldn't throw a baseball or a football. He only played a little catch with me when I was young.

My father was a moderate man: no madness possessed him; no crazy streak marked him; no passion distinguished him. His feelings showed most when he lost or won at cards, when drivers cut him off, or when someone miscalculated his bills. He never once bought a car he couldn't afford. He never saw the economics of growing a garden. Now, possibly at the threshold of my own death, I begrudged him the risks he never took, the passions he never generated, the strictures that held firm along the road of duty and obligation. He never taught me how to jump and sing.

Cleaning and tidying up were the ways my father imposed order on the world. He hung up his clothes as soon as he came home from work. He kept his closet in perfect order and always straightened the money in his wallet. He never did yard- or housework without putting on work clothes. He went about things rapidly—lickety-split was the word for his approach to work and cleaning. Outside he changed the screens and storm windows as the seasons required; he always had the right brushes and brooms for cleaning the screen and scraping the wood, and the proper sponge and chamois to clean the glass. He also had a large industrial broom he used for the garage and the sidewalk. He applied a second coat to everything he painted.

My mother admits that keeping my neat and tidy father clean—a white-collar worker at Western Union from the time he was sixteen until he retired—was not a hard job. Of course, she regularly washed and ironed his clothes, took his suits to the cleaners, and occasionally moved a button (always out rather than in) and darned a stocking or two. Compared to the neighborhood factory workers who kept the arsenal of democracy working around the clock, he was as clean as a whistle. Furthermore, he liked new clothes and shoes—near the end of his life he had a closet full of both. He took a bath twice a week and didn't need deodorant, and my mother claimed that his feet didn't stink like hers and her side of the family. He also didn't have dandruff, although he enjoyed the weekly shampoo my mother gave him.

My father treated the world like a set of pressing chores. As soon as he came home, he changed into his work clothes, ate rapidly (he ate quicker than any man alive and never said he enjoyed a meal, even though he usually did), and did what yardwork, house repairs, and book work were required. Then, unless he needed to run an errand or pay bills, he sat down for the rest of the evening to read the paper, do the crossword puzzle, and watch or listen to a ball game. Sometimes he listened to baseball while watching football. He went to bed around ten o'clock after sitting an hour or two in his easy chair, never understanding why he didn't sleep well.

His weekends (which in middle age included trips out into the country to buy fresh fruits or eat meals) increasingly resembled the rest of the week except that he attended mass and listened to more sports, and shopped for groceries. The holidays and frequent weddings, baptisms, and funerals provided some variation to his habitual order. Even the vacations he took when he was younger involved the family. We often took along my grandmother Amato and once my widowed Aunt Milly. Trips were like everything else. They were carefully planned, mapped, and measured in mileage and gasoline consumption. My dad prided himself on how many miles we covered in how many hours and days rather than enjoying anything we saw along the way. On this count he was not different from my uncles.

My dad was not a humorless man, but he didn't use irony, was never sarcastic, and rarely told a joke. He didn't speak off color. In fact, he once corrected me when I was young for saying "Nuts." As I grew older, I often felt he was drowning in my mother's unending stories of her childhood. But she added spice and fantasy to his matter-of-fact world.

My father worked and lived for the family. He worked to eat and ate to work. He did not live for opportunities and pleasures. The son of Sicilian mountain peasants, he was raised on the strict discipline of family and work.

My dad indulged himself modestly. He smoked a pipe for twenty years, from his late twenties to his late forties. He drank but never excessively, in his forties rarely more than one beer or glass of wine at a time. He did the crossword puzzle daily. He would pick it up again and again, in between periods of attention to the ball game on the radio or television, until he completed it or went to bed. He couldn't sing at all, although he enjoyed bellowing out hymns in church. He never went out of his way to listen to music, although he did have a soft spot for the sound of big bands, to which he and my mother danced, and he did like a well-sung Italian aria. He stood silently by when my mother went on a Mitch Miller rampage in the late 1950s. With the help of dozens of albums and their first record player, which came along with their new television, she kept the house in heavily overlain harmony. She subjected every visitor to an obligatory fifteen minutes of listening to "Those Wedding Bells Are Breaking Up That Old Gang of Mine" and other oldies but goodies.

My dad was a great sports fan. Round by round, fight by fight, he rooted for both the fine Italian and Detroit boxers. (I don't know what he would have done if Rocky Marciano had ever fought Joe Lewis.) He rooted for all Detroit sports teams — the Lions, the Red Wings, and especially his beloved Tigers. When I enrolled at the University of Michigan, he became an ardent "Go Blue!" fan. When I was a student, I brought him up to an occasional game. On one visit he was delighted when we came across the Michigan band practicing its half-time show number "Sing! Sing! Sing!" with none other than the great drummer, Gene Krupa.

After years of his loyally cheering the U of M's football and basketball teams, it seemed appropriate that he died listening to the final game of Michigan's successful bid for the 1989 national basketball championship. His death got mingled with the game in several ways.

I was watching the game in Minnesota, where I had settled with my family. I refused to take a long-distance call during the game until I was told that it concerned my father. The excitement of the close game had proved to be more than his heart could take. In one of my mother's several variations of the story, she said that my father took a glass of wine from her, asked her to open the window, told her he loved her, shouted "Go Blue!" and then turned blue and died. In any case, he died nearly instantly, watching a truly heart-stopping game.

Memories were hidden away in my father. Words were locked in his heart. He offered no flamboyant opinions. He told no stories; he did not speak with anecdotes. He proffered no subtle wisdom. He told me by his whole life that a person should do what they can and must. A person should not make too much or too little of himself.

Above all else, my dad was a counter. He kept numerical tabs of everything. He filled in the score card at ball games. Whenever we played cribbage, a game of counting, or pinochle, he kept score. He loved to mark things down. He was one of the few people I knew who faithfully and successfully kept lead in his mechanical pencils. He was always wrapping rubber bands around things, making small, neat packages of them. He used a lot of staples and paper clips to organize his papers. He put a lot of other small things in little boxes. He even had a couple of those dimpled rubber index finger covers for counting papers. In one of my favorite photographs of him, he is wearing a green visor, the kind businessmen and card players used to wear. He looks quizzically up at a Western Union messenger who, with a towel wrapped around his jaw, is asking if he can leave work to go to the dentist, which manifestly belied the two game tickets he held in his hand for the Detroit Tigers-Cleveland Indians opening game at Briggs Stadium.

His work spaces showed the same order as his files and drawers. He kept his paint brushes clean and sorted and stored in an old shoe bag. He kept his wrenches and other tools oiled. They were carefully hung above the tool bench he had built. He had an anvil, which was a foot section of city streetcar track, that he used for straightening nails, which he kept along with screws in little bins and baby food jars.

My father, who tallied so well, was manager of the union's credit union. Yet his conservatism kept him essentially out of the stock market. (The majority of stocks he bought were in Western Union, his employer.) As could be guessed, my dad bargained hard. This talent showed most when he shopped for cars. Starting after the Second World War, he and my uncles all bought new cars—always a Chevy, Plymouth, or Dodge—every three or four years. For two to three weeks before buying he would tour and telephone east-side car dealers, playing salesman off salesman, seeking their bedrock bottom price. Then, if my mother was satisfied with the color, he would bargain for an additional accessory or two, finally concluding the deal when the salesman conceded a free undercoating.

My father bargained in other areas as well. Most of the sales people with whom he worked were out of their league. They were dealing with the son of immigrants who had started selling fruit from a wagon when he was seven and began working at the Italian store at Eastern Market when he was twelve.

Although my father counted carefully, he wasn't cheap. He always paid his share when my parents went out. He treated anyone who came to the house generously, and he gave my mother wide latitude in buying whatever she wanted.

In comparison with my uncles, all of whom went to war, my dad's adventures centered on work and unions. He mastered job after job given him at the company and held every office in his union. His first adventures were about forming unions; later they were about personnel problems, odd management decisions, occasional holdups, and such episodes as spending the 1943 Detroit race riot near one of its epicenters at Western Union's downtown office.

He rarely went out, except to visit relatives, and almost never without my mother. My dad didn't have a group of men friends who hung together. He stayed at home. He belonged to no clubs, although he sat on the parish council and managed the co-op housing board. He engaged in no politics, even though his adherence to the Democratic Party and the advance of the working class never wavered. He didn't forget the party that had helped his family and his union in bad times.

My father never agonized over who he was or what he was to do. He never openly philosophized about what it meant to be the son of a poor immigrant family in a rich nation, or what he experienced in the process of making himself a Detroiter and an American. In contrast to me, he never struggled to become something, to bridge himself from one set of ideas or identity to another. He was confident about who he was and what actions were demanded by his situation. Remembering him—this good-natured and methodical man—offered me no consolation other than that I should do what I thought right, and he would love me whatever its outcome.

As he aged, however, he became more nervous. He turned small tasks into pressing obligations. And the older he got, the louder he got. He moaned more and more at cards. Though he played with only dimes and quarters, he cried out as if God should reconsider his plight. He sang even louder in church and grew more blunt in his expression. Shaking a man's coarse hand to whom he had just been introduced in our church basement, he blurted out, "I can see you are a farmer." He told a salesman that the product before him was as "useless as a crochet piss pot." On the church steps, he instructed the assembled local

Knights of Columbus, dressed in their full regalia of capes, admiral caps, and swords, "That way to the Falkland Islands!"

My father didn't want much from the world. He conformed to it and didn't expect others to rise above it. He didn't pick fights or hold grudges. He wasn't jealous or resentful. Nor was he a milquetoast. In fact, my dad stood for principles. He could get testy in battles and put up a tenacious fight. In his sixties, he took on the state unemployment office and beat them several times as they tried to whittle his compensation down to nothing. And until he died he was more than a handful for any billing officials who presumed they could outcount or outreason him.

His interior life always seemed hidden within himself or veiled by the excesses of my mother's ways. He rarely complained that she never let simple things be simple. Whatever caught her attention—a person, a store, a hobby—could quickly become a mania with her. For a few years in their middle forties, square dancing caught her fancy, and my dad was dressed in cowboy shirts and long string bow ties and, along with Uncle Bill and Aunt Margaret, dragged from one eastside gym to another. Only when the dancing reached the frequency of three nights a week did my father openly resist, on the grounds of sore muscles and having to work the next day. I was glad. For my father to become an American was one thing; to be a Sicilian peasant transformed into a singing and dancing cowboy was another.

My mom seldom dropped a subject once she started on it. She would endlessly repeat stories from her childhood. At such times, my exasperated father would say: "She remembers everything, and I, nothing."

I wished he would have found a way to defy her and the duties that tethered him to a staid life. But such a rebellion would never have fit him. He was sequestered by the life he and my mother had chosen to live. He subdued her by not letting her work or have more children, and she domesticated him by not allowing him to circle too far from home (which he never wanted to do anyway). They obeyed the limits they embraced. They resisted change, and won. In my mind I went back and forth, blaming each for not living the lives I hoped for them and myself.

Most of all, I wished my dad would have lent his imagination to his own future. He could have easily been a lawyer, an accountant, or a political leader. Or, I wanted him to learn to shirk his duty—to take long weekends for fishing, hunting, or golf. But that was not him. He was as determined in his ways as any peasant. There was a grim integrity about his life that he uncharacteristically contradicted, just after I had gotten married, by telling me, "Have a good time. Life goes by quickly."

Now, at his graveside, I no longer felt a need to argue with him. I simply regretted that our hearts had not drawn closer together. I wished I had told him more often how much I loved him and what a good father he was. I wished I had openly asked him for help when I needed it, and I wished I had tried harder to persuade him to take up golf or skating so we could have shared the pleasures I've shared with my sons and daughters.

We did have our good hours together. We drank beer, played bocce ball, went to a Tigers game, prayed shoulder to shoulder in church, agreed that Republicans aren't our kind of people, and argued over what was worst about our shared Democratic Party. We each knew—and there is a dignity in knowing this—that in some unalterable way fathers and sons are not meant to be soul mates. They are not meant to be nose to nose, heart to heart, on this earth.

Standing at his grave, I knew we were joined in loyalty to work and family. And I sensed, with my bypass pending, that, if heaven made any human sense, we would be joined in life after death. I remembered once watching him asleep in his recliner, which he did more frequently during the last years of his life, and writing a poem.

A Sicilian Father

My father appears to be practicing dying.
He is reclined in his recliner.
His face is long and drawn, ashen white,
His breath,
Deep,
Precarious,
Hesitant.
He goes
Where no living man dares.

Like every son
I am drawn to and driven from

My sleeping father.
He is all I am, all I fear.
Fleeing him,

I follow the circle of things,
I go to the land
Of his father and mother.

In Sicily,
At the Greek temple Segesta
(raised seven centuries before Christ),
I observe how snails,
Circular temples themselves,
Once alive,
Now decorate the dead, bleached-white stems
Of bent, scattered plants.

Small brown birds
Fly in and out
Of the roofless, half-standing temple,
Building nests on its highest ledges.

I follow a shepherd and his flock higher up,
To the amphitheater that surveys the land and sea below.
I sit on the highest row of curved stone.
Among grazing sheep,
I ask what tragedies
Fed ancient Sicilians.

My father left me keeper of the graves. I knew that as long as

I lived my heart would be the temple of the family dead—I would keep the memory of their lives; I'd not forget their hopes and sacrifices; I would pray for them. And if I am destined to die, I thought, perhaps we will soon have the conversation we both deserve. We might even dance and sing a bit, too.

I left his grave, as he would have me, to visit those of his parents.

Broken Journeys

I found my father's parents' graves by locating the black stone monument dedicated to the prominent east-side Calcaterra family. Their graves stood on a knoll, in the shadow of a small tree, alongside the graves of my dad's sister, Fina, and her husband, Phil. I found them partially sunk and covered by grass, obviously untended since I was there last. My dad had always brought along to the cemetery a little bucket, a small collapsible World War II trench shovel, and a garden trowel with which to tend the graves. I used my pocket knife to cut away the thick tufts of grass that covered their names.

My grandfather, Antonino Amato, died in 1915 of appendicitis when he was thirty-three. One day on the way to work his appendix ruptured. The next day he was dead. My grandmother, Rosalia, was left alone with my three-year-old father and his newly born infant sister, Fina. My grandfather's abrupt death concealed him from us. At his graveside, thoughts of his premature death blocked any self-pity on my part. Even if I were to die in the days ahead, I would have already lived out the greater portion of my life and completed much of what I started, while he was cut down in his prime, at the very beginning of his journey into marriage, America, and a life of his own making.

My father never knew him, and he spurned reflecting on it as much as my mother constantly dwells on and reinvents the past. My father was never interested in prying apart the things that are with thoughts about what might or might not have been. He never once mentioned his father to me, leaving him a puzzle for me to piece together.

In the small coal town of Kelayres, Pennsylvania, where my family first arrived when they emigrated from the old country and where I still have cousins, I met an old schoolteacher, Tony DiMaria, who knew my grandfather. Tony, nearing ninety and complaining about ill-fitting shoes— *"Questi scarpi mi fannu male"*— told me stories about the early Sicilians of Kelayres. With unusual gusto he told about one old-timer who grew tired of Irish baseball players chasing pop flies into his garden. He went in his house, retrieved a pistol he had brought from the old country, and returned to the field and shot the catcher and the pitcher in the leg. He wasn't arrested, and thereafter a number of fly balls lay untouched in his garden. Unfortunately, Tony had no such stories to tell of my grandfather; he knew only that Antonino worked in the grocery store for a while.

At his graveside I thought how lucky I was to be spared an old Sicilian fate—not to be killed by appendicitis at a young age, and in all likelihood to survive open-heart surgery in middle life. Not expecting an answer, but revealing the way my mind worked, I wondered at his graveside whether one family member's misfortune assures another member's good fortune. Did Antonino's early death somehow add to my longevity? Yet my urge to have this question answered in the affirmative ran smack into my strong sense that suffering attracts suffering. I thought of cursed families, in which membership assured tragedy. Still, I persisted in believing that a personal God allows one family member's tragedies to ransom another's future suffering. After all, didn't God alter the entire course of history in response to his son's crucifixion?

Such reflections didn't bring me an inch closer to my grandfather, that short, handsome, square-shouldered and strong-jawed young man whose photograph, along with candles, crochet doilies, and the Infant of Prague had turned my grandmother's dresser top into a shrine. The dead were never far off in our family.

Beyond the photograph, Antonino is for me little more than conjecture about one of those countless Sicilian mountain peasants who left the old world for the new. I envision a young man who came down out of the Madonie Mountains in search of a better life. He knew if he stayed at home he would at best work to eat and eat to work, and know nothing more until he died. He would not have a horse or a mule, perhaps only a donkey, a few small tracts of land, with a few vines, olive trees, a field of *carciofi* (artichokes), and a garden. He would have had to scrape a living off the land or out of his native village, Cerda. Before deciding to leave he must have weighed the conflicting truths of two proverbs. His fears must have said, "He who leaves the old way for the new knows what he is losing but not what he will find *(Che lascia la via vecchia per la nuova, sa quel que perde e non sa quel que trova).* His common sense probably argued that to stay here in these mountains is to have nothing, and, in the words of a second proverb, "He who hasn't, isn't" *(Chi non a, non è).* Yielding to the latter, he must have concluded that to stay in Cerda would be to remain a nobody.

I know from my grandmother that he came directly from Cerda to an even smaller American village, Kelayres, in the hard-coal region of Pennsylvania, where he joined a brother and a sister. He worked in the mines a single day — at the end of which he vowed never to return to the toil and darkness below. A few years of work in a grocery store gave him sufficient means to marry my grandmother, his brother-in-law's sister.

The sixteen-year-old bride, Rosalia Notaro, who only a few years before had traveled alone from Montemaggiore Belsito, a village at the very top of the valley of the Madonie Mountains, was quick to conceive. Believing claims that things were better in Detroit, where new industries were expanding at an extraordinary rate in the first decade of the century, Antonino took his family there in 1911. He, along with thousands of new migrants from the east, arrived too late. Factory production was down; the first burst of expansion was over. He could find only odd jobs and irregular work. On one occasion, frequently described by my grandmother, he went to Ford Motor for employment and there, while waiting for work, underwent the humiliating experience, along with hundreds of other job seekers, of being driven away from the premises of Ford Motors in Dearborn by men armed with fire hoses.

My grandmother told me that, when they were first married, my grandfather insisted on making love as soon as he returned home from work. In their embrace, I assume, they found the warmth and joy so absent from their daily toil. Perhaps they sensed the family and village they had left behind and found the energy to venture forward into this strange world.

What little headway they had made in their new life was radically cut short when Antonino died. He had not been given time to realize the fruits of his migration. His first son, born in 1909 and also named Joseph, as my father was, had been scalded to death when he upset a bucket of scrub water on himself. My father and Fina were mere infants. He was still a long way from the village he sought in the United States of America. He never made it to the blessed age when a retired immigrant sits (as so many have in Detroit and across the nation) on the front porch of his own home, surely worn but content and proud, knowing that he made a family, bought a home of his own, and so bent the world to his will.

The young couple's crossing was aborted; tragedy had not been left behind. Antonino was dead. Rosalia's heart was broken, and she put on the black dress she wore for the rest of her days. It fell to her to carry on. Alone with two children, my father and Fina, her only support was what consolation her prayers could bring and what counsel and aid a married brother and sister and a few friends, especially her *cumari*, the Brucatos, gave her.

After a few years she remarried, and from that marriage came three more daughters, Josephine, Milly, and Pauline. The man she had married abused Fina. Doing what no one in the old country would have done, she took him to court, and he was sentenced to jail for at least fifteen years. I was about ten when I first met him. He gave me a gift of a large hunting knife with a purple plastic handle. It was as intimidating as it was ugly. The only other time I ever saw him was one Memorial Day. He stood at a corner of Mount Olivet Cemetery selling small American flags and other grave decorations.

Spoiled for marriage by her violation, Fina was given in marriage to Phil, an older Sicilian and a good man for whom I always had a lot of affection. Fina died near the end of the Second World War midway through her first pregnancy when a blood clot went to her brain. Several years later, Phil, whom we considered part of the family, returned to the old country for a bride. With her—an older, not very intelligent or good-looking woman—he had and raised two children in what year by year became an increasingly run-down and crime-filled neighborhood. Our families grew steadily apart until we only heard of Phil secondhand. The news was never good. We heard he was having trouble raising his children. Finally, we heard that he had died after a long period of mental disorganization during which he suffered fits in which he believed that the Mafia was out to get him. The last I heard, his wife and two children moved to Wisconsin thirty years or so ago where she had relatives. Apparently, they hadn't returned to Phil's grass-covered grave for a long time. Clearly, Phil and my grandmother had not left *la miseria* behind in Sicily.

I—baseball player, golfer, student at the University of Michigan, teacher—was always close to Rosalia, my grandmother

Amato. I never doubted that she loved me. She was a short, heavy woman, 4' 6", weighing nearly 180 pounds. I took her size, along with her quick temper, wonderful breaded veal, and generous Christmas and birthday gifts, as natural. Not until I was older did I realize the burden she carried.

I remember her in the house my father bought for her on Hilger Avenue on the east side. The surrounding frame houses (now either torn down or surrounded by fields of high weeds or industrial parking lots) harbored people of all ages and nationalities. In the duplex next door lived a noisy Greek family with a boy my age who was a good left-handed pitcher. Two blocks over were our cousins, the De Carlos, my grandmother's sister Pauline and her husband Joe, who made good wine and buried and resurrected his fig tree each year. They had four sons: Joe, the oldest, loudest, thus most authoritative son; Andy, smooth-voiced and friendly, the natural salesman; and Steve, raucous, good-natured, and entrepreneurial, and eventual owner of his own machine shop. They were my father's first cousins and friends, especially Steve and Andy. And there was the youngest, Paul, my godfather, a short, kind man and a well-known east-side music instructor, who had a little mustache that I never liked, and who, during the war, played the accordion rather than carry a weapon. All of the De Carlo boys were dead, and even two of Andy's children: his oldest boy, Guy, and second son, Paul, my friend and godfather to my daughter Felice. Death was seeping into my generation.

Fina and Phil lived a block over. Phil loved pinochle and had a terraced garden along one side of his small lot. When I went to their house I was always fussed over and given a lot to eat. I was amazed by the way Phil held his cards like the fancy tail of a bird. Across the street from grandmother's was her brother, Uncle John. In my memory, John—Cruciano, his Italian name—never spoke. He seemed as distant as he was silent. I saw him all summer long, hunched over and head bent, tirelessly hoeing his garden. As if to balance out his silence, his wife, Margaret, my grandfather's sister, was gregarious, loud, and gravel-voiced. She could easily be heard from across the street when she was out on her front porch. Detroit may have been a rising industrial city, but my dad's family, like so many others, formed a peasant village under the shadows of Chrysler Motors.

When I was at my grandmother's, which was usually Sunday afternoons, things were always astir. My dad's three sisters scurried about. First they were unmarried, then accompanied by boyfriends, and then married with children of their own. The war marched in and out of grandmother's house as well. Josephine's husband, Jimmy, sold his car, went off to war in the infantry, and before being shipped out had a photograph of himself taken in a studio against a jungle background: Crouched, with his legs spread far apart, he held a giant knife in his right hand. Danny, the tall sailor from Texas, visited my Aunt Milly. My cousin Angel (Josephine and Jimmy's daughter) and I waited to spy his long stride coming down Hilger from distant Mack Avenue. When he finally arrived, announced in advance by me and my cousin, he and Milly hugged on the couch in the front room all afternoon.

The heart of the house was the round dining room table at which we ate and celebrated and the kitchen with its ice box, window box, table, and stove. Food formed the center of home. In the closets and bathtub pots of beans were set to soak. In the basement there was an occasional chicken in a cage, along with a wine barrel. My grandmother knew how to wring the chickens' necks and scald off their feathers. Under her bed there was a two-foot-long box of spaghetti. Individual noodles made excellent swords, which I would eat when they snapped off in battle.

My grandmother animated the household during the day. Angel and I cringed in the face of her stern defense of the living room and household goods. But for every scolding she gave me, she compensated me—the first-born son of her only son, born of her first husband—with hugs and money. During the night I would snuggle up to sleep next to her. In the morning I would take pride in listening to her tell my parents how my kicking and turning had kept her awake much of the night.

I recall the moments when my grandmother was happy. She loved our short Sunday trips into the countryside; they provided an occasion to stop and buy fruit and to reminisce about the riches of Sicily. And until later in life, she enjoyed longer trips to northern Michigan, Wisconsin, and once to Florida. They were a way to forget some things and to be part of our family—to be with her son, Joe, his wife Ethel (*Etella*), and her only grandson, Joey. Sometimes during these trips she became almost as spontaneous as a child. I remember once in particular when my parents hired a buggy to tour Mackinaw Island. My grandmother and I had the honor of sitting up front, directly behind the driver and his farting horse. With each step, a fart; with each fart, a laugh. Old forts, other historic sights, and the Grand Hotel itself faded into the background, and it seemed as if the island itself shook amid our laughter.

Even in the last years of her life a brief trip to the Italian store was enough to animate her. It was as if she had returned to the foods and ways of her childhood. But for all the times I saw her happy, there are countering images of sadness. For every time I saw her dance at a wedding, I saw her weep at a funeral. For every time I remember her happy in her kitchen, I recall her afflicted with pain—especially as she walked slowly out of the school where she worked as a janitor, complaining how hard and heavy her work was. Once, quite by accident, she got on a bus I was riding, and several minutes passed before I recognized the short, worn woman dressed in black at the front of the bus as my grandmother.

I don't know when I first began to sense the tragic in her life. Perhaps it was when I got old enough to sense the tragic in life itself. Perhaps it was when she began to cough uncontrollably, until she often wet herself, and even then she couldn't stop coughing. But the tragic had been there since the heartbreak of the loss of her first love, Antonino. She had come from another world, had lived another life, and was always close to welcoming death. She was forever in need of what love we gave her. Long before she died, the graveyard (*il camposanto*) had a strong hold on her. It contained Tony, their first son, my dad's sister Fina, and even young and lovable Sam, who returned home from the war—like Jimmy he fought in the Italian campaign—married Milly, and five years later died after a long and miserable bout with stomach cancer. Lying in the bed where my grandmother and I had slept, Sam wasted away, casting an ever larger shadow over the home and family. I never forgot Sam's long and slow death; in a twisted way, it consoled me for having a faulty heart and having to undergo the risk of cardiac surgery.

At a certain point, death alone promised the rendezvous she cherished. The last ten years of her life were heavy with pain. She moved from the old neighborhood with Aunt Mildred and her second husband, Dale, to the far east side of Detroit, where the Italians had not yet fully reassembled themselves with stores and church communities. Sequestered by age, culture, and circumstances, there wasn't much for my grandmother to do but wait for death and argue with Milly, whom when angry she accused of being a no-good whore, as only a Mediterranean mother can. Visits from the relatives, biweekly trips to the Italian store, fresh supplies of fruit, and a few outing to weddings and funerals weren't enough to reverse her destiny. Afflicted with emphysema, she turned more and more to asking God for death. And in her final hours, when I stood vigil down the hall, I too prayed that her belabored breathing would stop. She had journeyed far enough. She deserved a rest, a sleep that would free her from *la miseria*. That alone might reunite her with her Antonino and satisfy the dreams and hopes of this peasant girl from the Madonie Mountains.

At her graveside, broken crossings—failed bypasses—preoccupied my mind. The distance between what was desired and what was granted loomed large. A successful bypass was no certainty. Prayer was not a sure bridge for earthly hopes.

Perhaps I would fall between the cracks of life, as so many in my family had.

⌒═══⌒

My grandmother Amato's life stood in sharp contrast to the lives of my grandmother and grandfather Linsdau. I always reflected on the differences when I drove from her home to theirs or when I walked from her grave to theirs. After a short stop and prayer at the nearby graves of Sam and my great aunt May—a World War One nurse and my mother's favorite aunt—I left the old, wooded part of the cemetery for the new, flat, treeless section, where my grandparents Linsdau were buried.

My grandmother Amato's crossing had been shattered en route. Theirs had remained intact. She had lived most of her life without a husband; they had been married for more than fifty years. When she came to this country to begin a new life, my grandparents' parents—from Germany, Ireland, and elsewhere—had already established themselves in the new land. In my mind, she was my Italian grandparent, and they, though themselves the children of relatively recent immigrants, were my American grandparents.

My grandfather's father, Jakob Linsdau, was a bar carver from Alsace-Lorraine. He came to Milwaukee, worked in the Fox River Valley, and then settled in Menasha. There he married an Irish girl named Mary Jane O'Brien. He opened a saloon, even though Mary Jane was adamantly against drink, accumulated some wealth, and served as a Menasha alderman. The family had their own pew near the front of the church, and a noisy band played at his funeral.

My grandmother Linsdau's father, Boodry, a Scotch Presby-
terian whom I in appearance so resemble, came to Wisconsin
from out east. He married a Protestant girl with the English
name of Sayre when he was fourteen and she was twelve. He
was a teamster and then a veterinary assistant until he died of a
rabid dog bite in his forties. Nothing could be done for him.
My grandmother, Frances, who never lacked for a melodra-
matic story, told me that he began to snap at people. His friends
tied him down, blindfolded him, and shot him to death.
Decades later, a cousin told me that they had intended to shoot
him if he had another convulsion, which he didn't. It occurred
to me that, surrounded as I would be by doctors, nurses, and
machines, my death would be gentle compared to his.

My grandmother Amato's stories were Sicilian—about leading a donkey up into the mountains, the snake that barred her
way into the olive orchard, the prince of Montemaggiore Belsito who threw coins out of his carriage. In contrast, my grandmother and grandfather Linsdau's stories were American: they
had the scent of Tom Sawyer and Huck Finn about them. They
were always on the way up north, near lakes, on the banks of a
creek, or up in the woods. They spoke of rolling hoops; paint-
ing cows and tipping over outhouses as Halloween pranks; and
going squirrel hunting. They told me how to remove the curse
from a white horse and make wishes come true by placing a
chip of wood over your spit on the ground. They described
haunted houses in their Wisconsin towns and one local church
to which each night a priest revenant returned to say his
uncompleted masses. They told many stories of weddings,

bands, dances, and failed romances that ended in pregnancy and suicide. They told tales of their own relatives. There was Aunt Sade, a recluse who often pretended she was not home, but whose presence in the winter was revealed by footprints in the snow leading to the outhouse. And there was my grandfather's brother, Emmett, who performed in vaudeville and dabbled in photography, and one day walked downtown nude carrying an umbrella. There was grandpa Linsdau's parrot, given to him when the bird's antiphone to the Our Father and Hail Mary were corrupted by vulgarisms taught to it by school children. Jakob took the corrupted parrot in—but much to his dismay the ingrate parrot got in the habit of announcing "Pa is leaving" every time Jake left his upstairs apartment for the bar he owned below. Even when Jake covered his cage before trying to make his escape, the foulmouthed parrot would respond to the sound of squeaking stairs with "Pa is leaving!"

Unlike my grandmother Amato, whose clear fate and fixed emotions told her who she was, my grandmother Linsdau was always in search of herself. Her heart was never sure of itself; her moods were strong; her mind was always peripatetic. She always stood between two opposite worlds. She espied relief elsewhere, and her desires led her away from others. Life was no easy crossing for her. As I grew older and struggled to find my own identity, I felt that her restless spirit had passed into me. Up to her last years in life, she spoke to me as a kindred spirit. She correctly connected my going to college with thinking and feeling and writing about life's deepest matters. She shared her regrets over missed educational opportunities—surely a year of business school had not been enough for her — and she often insisted that one day she would write a book of recollections.

Within Grandma Linsdau's spirit resided many people. Her sensibility embraced, at one and the same time, the Presbyterianism of her youth and the Catholicism to which she converted when she married my grandfather. She identified with poets and songwriters. She balanced (not unlike the great Jean-Jacques Rousseau himself) between a profound desire to shine in the eyes of others and an equally strong wish to remove herself as far as possible from the fixing glance of society. She was spared knowledge of her divided self by the obedient love of my grandfather, who slavishly catered to her whims, moving her from house to house, place to place, when it sometimes cost him promotions and even jobs.

Her changing self led her down two separate paths. She wanted unswerving allegiance from others and, consequently, followed the heart-rending cycle of enthusiastically embracing another person as a dear friend, then quickly coming to expect too much from that person, becoming angry, and hoping never to see the person again. Sometimes, in a matter of weeks, my grandmother would move into a new house, praise the neighbors, damn the neighbors, and drive my grandfather to sell the house and move again. At times, she even turned her demand for loyalty into playing favorites among her children. Once I even saw her, eyes crazy with fear and accusation, challenge my grandfather's fidelity to her.

There was something terribly modern about the whirl of her cravings. Inside the devoted mother who raised three children

(Ethel, Mabel, and Bill) and who cooked great meal after great meal for nearly sixty years, there was a restless woman who moved her itinerant family from house to house, apartment to cottage, city to countryside, and back again. She made over thirty moves in all. My mother never stayed in the same school for more than two years. Within this woman who could play cards by the hour (until her grandson was unable to distinguish hearts from clubs), who could take three nights of bingo a week, ten cards at a time (leaving the characters "B-7" indelibly written on her grandson's mind), who could sit in a boat fishing from nearly sunup to sundown (until her grandson began to see drowning as a relief), there was a soul in search of a self, a place, a reassuring order of things. Poetry (rather dark and sentimental), tales of vendetta and suicide (unduly morbid), and philosophizing (cogent and generous at times) expressed a soul that was no longer anchored in the collectivity of the old world and not yet comfortable in the individuality of the new. I came to know her madness, for in measure it resided in my mother and me—and in every person. The older I grew the more determined I was not to allow her spirit to gallop loose in me.

A few years before she died, she returned home from a secondhand store with two books for me. One was a collection of poetry; the other was titled *The Great Hereafter, or Glimpses of the Coming World*. She wanted me to remember her in my future reflections as the grandmother who was interested in the meaning of life.

Death came long and hard for her as a series of strokes, none mortal, each debilitating, weakening her over a number of years.

In contrast to Grandmother Amato's suffering over how things had been, Grandma Linsdau's anguish was about how things might have been.

The contrast between Grandpa and Grandma Linsdau could not have been more extreme. It amounted to nothing other than the difference between a heavy and a light spirit. My Grandpa Linsdau lived by a wisdom different from everyone else's in the family. At least, it seemed so to me, the grandson whom he taught to shoot a slingshot and a .22 rifle, and for whom he always had a joke or a bizarre story to tell, or something he was working on in the basement or garage to show. He always had time for a game of pool or croquet.

The armor of his humor did not crack until his very last years, when he had lost his wife and suffered heart attacks and strokes. Until then, it seemed to me that he had set his sails in invisible winds that moved him out of the troublesome waters that beat against most people. To walk a dog, play a harmonica, listen to a ball game, tend a garden, say an evening prayer — whatever was simple — seemed to suffice. In his magic world he made little things matter a lot. He fit all that was playful and innocent in my childhood.

At his house there was always a chance to play. There was rummy and a lot of pencil-and-paper games like tic-tac-toe, hangman, and COOTIE. More fun yet were slingshots and stilts to be made and used. My grandfather was a crack shot, and he could walk up and down stairs on stilts. On special occasions we would try out his .22 rifle. One of my first shots, when I was five, went through my cousin's doll buggy and a five-gallon jug of linseed oil in his garage. It served him with a good story for decades. He always sought to be amusing. When I visited him in my twenties, he would insist that I say "Hello" to his dog and that his dog reply with a bark before I could cross the threshold from his porch into his living room. After that I was required to have a shot and a beer before we settled down to a three-game pool tournament.

When I was young, I wanted to have large-veined, knowing hands like his. He made and did things with them that I wished I could. He hoed expansive gardens, built rock chimneys, and took porcupine quills out of my dog's face. My adoring eyes didn't notice that he had a glass eye (lost when a boy) until my mother told me. I didn't question his obedient love for my grandmother. I also didn't know just how sentimental and soft-hearted he was until my mother told me that when her three-year-old baby sister Ellen died, Grandpa Linsdau was inconsolable. Brokenhearted, he aimlessly wandered about town for months, visiting her grave every day. I never attributed a mean side to him even when I heard his harsh opinions on those he didn't agree with, which seemed to grow in reaction to the protest of the 1960s, or when he told me how he shot dogs from his porch with a slingshot or put fish hooks in the pea patch to catch sparrows and starlings. He was my grandfather and friend.

He always seemed to be on stage. He put on the women's hats at Easter, danced an odd jig when the music was right, and tickled more than one person when they weren't looking. To the boss or bully (or somebody who just rubbed him wrong) he was quick to use his favorite phrase: "Kiss my ass!" Toward most people he was kind. And to those he knew best he was lovable and, at times, a damnable tease, inventing names and telling stories. He nicknamed one of my uncles, a high school track star, "drag ass," claiming that his short legs and low-slung behind allowed him to spark himself into high speed. Before my dad married my mother, he was not generous in his comments on Italians. At times he hunted down situations and caused embarrassments, especially to his young daughters when they were dating. Once he took a pair of his shoes and a pair of his daughter's and pressed them in the snow on the front porch to resemble the tracks of embracing lovers. Then he called his daughter out to see the footprints and upbraided her for such carrying on. He transformed some of his jokes into family traditions by repeating them over and over. He taught every one of his grandchildren how to skip the wrong way, making it a forward hop with one stiff, trailing leg. This caused my parents and uncles and aunts no end of grief with their children's kindergarten teachers, who had to enforce the public requirement that children know how to skip before they enter first grade. His improvisations, subtle and coarse, went on and on. They stopped just short of his father's trick of sending grandchildren chasing after farts with bags, offering them a nickel for each one they caught.

When grandmother died, grandfather Linsdau's health faltered. He wasn't made to live alone. He ate TV dinners, called his son and daughters frequently, and wouldn't let visitors leave. He was lonely, terribly lonely. He would cry openly and bitterly over the conditions life had reduced him to. Yet even during my last visit with him at his house, he tried hard to make me and my new bride, Cathy, laugh.

One day he forgot to light the oven and filled the house with gas, which caused him to have another stroke. After two days in a coma, he came to, only to find he couldn't speak any more. He sank back into a final coma and breathed heavily until he died.

I couldn't stand at his graveside without believing that we would be rejoined again—even if only for a blessed instant of mutual recognition, to express the love we shared. I found it difficult to believe we could survive death, or would care to survive it, without consciousness of those we love. It seemed like only yesterday my grandfather and I were together. He belonged to my heart. Our youths were joined—our boyhoods crossed with the pull of a slingshot. The irrational hope that we would be together again carried me far.

Boyhood Days

Bypass made me feel frail and precarious—a mere reed in the winds of time. I sensed myself to be the sole creation of a time, place, and particular set of circumstances. On the verge of oblivion, I strove to find the boy of whom I was an extension. To regain him—the deepest kernel of self—I needed to visit a friend. No richer source could be found to know the boy who was and still is me.

For that reason, I made plans to meet my friend Ron at 10:00 P.M. at a bar on Woodward Avenue between downtown and Wayne State University. On the way there, I drove through old neighborhoods and past favorite places to awaken memories. I would see and remember all that I could; nothing was too insignificant to be forgotten. With death riding on my shoulder, I would be the Buddha of the great way, remembering everything and everyone who came to mind. More simply, I would resurrect all I could to bid it a possible farewell.

I stopped at my old grade school and gazed at the gravel play yard. There my slides into home base had ended in nasty cuts and scrapes, and there, in winter, I had asserted my dominance as the fastest skater. From the grade school I drove down the road that we had pedaled back and forth on our bikes one summer on our way to an east-side championship in baseball. I hunted down the house of the girl I first seriously dated and drove the streets she and I had so infatuatedly traveled hand and hand. I was pervaded by all that I knew about her and the feelings about her that filled my soul then.

I knew memory could not defeat time. I conceded that God would do with us as he wished. Yet, I protested in advance: I didn't want my childhood surrendered to oblivion. I insisted that being—the entirety of things—would not end until certain broken or severed things could be repaired. I couldn't imagine crossing the threshold of eternity before again telling the girl I first loved that I truly loved her and receiving forgiveness for the love I could not reciprocate. If only for one revealing, loving glance, walls erected by whole lives must come down. God must shatter the kernel of ourselves.

I had sought out Ron because he was the key, in the words of Willa Cather, "to all those memories; one cannot get another set; one has but those." Ron and I got to know each other when our bodies were filling out, our senses were keenest, and impressions were freshest. We experienced many things together for the first time in our young lives. Free of past imprints, there is an immediacy and wholeness to the world of boyhood—which now felt so real to me with my present overrun by thoughts of pending surgery and my future suspended.

Together Ron and I went to the same grade school, Stellwagen on Outer Drive Avenue. He was a half year behind me. We had many of the same teachers, sat in the same rooms of the two-story English country-like school, heard the same buzzing alarm between classes, participated in the same mock fire drills and atomic attacks, stood at attention during the same flag ceremonies, ate the same government surplus apples, had the same friends, and together were amazed by our classmate Willy Bitta, who once hung out the window and another time threw scissors at the teacher before they hauled him off to reform school. We played on the same schoolyard, skated on the same ice pond, and played the same games behind the school. We gambled by flipping cards and pitching coins, played handball against the brick wall and metal grated window, and wrecked our bikes in our self-invented game of "bicycle derby." We played bicycle derby on a large elevated cement structure meant to receive coal. The object of the game was to force every other rider to touch the ground or the wall or drive them off the court. The winner, which I never once was, was the kid who stayed on his bike to the end. The ultimate loser, often a young kid with a brand-new bike, was the one who had to explain to his dad why his new bike's fenders were bent, spokes broken, or chain guard (a favorite place to kick) mashed in.

One spring evening, when we were in the eighth grade, Ron and I got in big trouble behind the school. One of us—I've forgotten which one—got the bright idea that with my dad's crowbar we could open the large grate adjacent to the bicycle derby court. We would then having free pickings of all the things at the bottom—balls, pencils, pens, baseball cards, and, better yet, pennies, nickels, dimes, and possibly a few quarters and fifty-cent pieces. Hardly had we emerged from the bottom of the grate with our haul and started to ride out of the darkening schoolyard than around the corner drove a police car, scouring the back of the school with its spotlight. They caught sight of us. We, as kids will, made a run for it. I threw away the crowbar and peddled as hard as I could. Ron took a clever turn to the right while I rode straight ahead. Yet the police followed him instead of me. They caught Ron and interrogated him. He didn't want to get hauled home to his sick mother, as the police threatened to do, unless he would tell them who I was. Ron persisted in his story that he just met me and didn't know my name. I sat at home awaiting the appearance of police officers at our front door. They never came. When I called Ron and discovered that he had not escaped, but still had refused to give them my name, my estimate of his friendship soared.

Ron and I first got to know each other outside of school in scouts. We hung together during weekends and the ten-day summer camp at a scout cabin on the Clinton River. We were under the order of the same scout master, A.J., a bachelor who had considered becoming a priest but instead dedicated his life to Troop 118, which assembled at our grade school. A.J.'s rule was tolerant; he endured us admirably. He only lost his temper when we turned his pancakes, of which he was so proud, into carp bait, bombarded with rocks the outdoor toilet in which he sat, and hid his punishing stick, which was an inch-thick wood street sign literally labeled "Bloody Road." We sealed it between the walls of a new addition to our cabin. A.J. couldn't play baseball well (he threw and batted "like a girl"), but he loved to play and made sure that we played. Our preference, even though our troop—to his pride—earned its share of life and eagle scouts (of which I was one) was to play with bull-whips, long hunting knives, and bows with thirty- and even forty-pound pulls, which we used for shooting carp. We made frequent trips into the woods, where we usually smoked cigarettes and once sickeningly chewed too much tobacco.

A.J. couldn't swim. This shortcoming kept him from attaining the rank of eagle scout, which he so coveted, until it was granted to him as an honor at the end of his scouting career. But he had the courage to let us swim. We dived off an old dock and swam through deep sheets of spring frog eggs and among water snakes to the opposite shore of the river, where we precariously stood on a slimy log shouting insults about cowardice at those who remained on the dock.

Once, Ron pushed me into the water to save a new scout who, yielding to the taunting of other scouts—"Sissy! Sissy!"—had jumped into the water over his head, even though he couldn't swim. Helplessly, frantically, he struggled his way to the surface, only to sink again, until Ron shoved me in with the command, "Save him!" I pulled the victim the few feet back to shore, for which he gave me candy and said I saved his life, even though I told him Ron really saved him.

A.J. did have rules. He required that we be on time for

meals, observe lights out, and never talk back. Until hidden away, "Bloody Road" was called into service for severe violations—and it did sting bitterly. However, his most severe discipline—at least it seemed to us, a true collection of all-American Tom Sawyers—was making us go to church every Sunday. But some scouts found a way around that obligation. No sooner were the Protestants dropped off at their church and our scout bus pulled away from the curb than our pious Protestant friends would walk right past the open church door and march over to the ice cream parlor. A.J. accompanied the rest of us to the long Catholic mass to whose bitter end he insisted we stay. An hour later, when we Catholics finally reached the ice cream parlor, we would find our Protestant friends already there, slyly smiling, drinking their second malted milks. I knew our religion was more serious than theirs.

At camp we hiked as far as our legs could carry us. "Keep Out! Private Property!" signs didn't stop us. In small groups, we wandered through stands of sumac, into lowlands, and even through itch weed and stinging nettles, if our imaginary warfare required it. We pushed the canoe into every back channel we could find and we rammed it into the rowboat, which usually held the younger and less noble scouts. Our greatest triumphs at camp were our canoe and rowboat wars. In our minds, we were quick and stealthy Indians pitted against the cumbersome strength of Roman galleons. We also tried filling the canoe with as many people as it would hold until it tipped. Once this trick almost cost me my life when my foot got caught up between the seat and the brace bar behind the seat. I escaped by rotating my whole body a half circle under the submerged canoe. That was the second time in my life I came close to drowning. The other time, I slid off my Aunt Mable's moss-covered dock and almost drowned in front of my grandparents until a boy grabbed me and pulled me out of the water. I had always considered myself a candidate for death by drowning. I never thought that one day my heart might fail me.

Winter meant other types of dangerous explorations at scout camp. We loved to establish at whim new tobogganing trails. They always led to spills, and once and a while they led smack into small trees and buried ice floes. Only the short length of the hills on the banks of the river saved me and the others from broken legs and necks. In early winter, we probed the river to test how well it was frozen. Usually it wasn't frozen as deep as our curiosity was long. One winter we pulled several boys from the water who had broken through. Another time my friend Doug went through the ice where the spring entered the river. No sooner had he taunted us, "Come on, you chickens!" than down he went through the soft ice into the river. Good swimmer that he was, he barely saved himself from the deep water, while we stood by and laughed.

Everything we did then went so vividly, so fresh to our hearts. Body and mind shared a state of wonderful simultaneity. Boyhood freely took everything to heart. It was about finding a bird's nest or a snake hole, catching frogs, collecting tadpoles, putting out grass fires, playing tug-of-war, sleeping outdoors in lean-tos made of saplings and sumac branches, and eating our own cooking (a restrictive cuisine that usually amounted to hunter's stew and baked potatoes, followed by roasted marshmallows).

Healthy boys that we were, camp involved us in continual tests of strength and skill. We stuck knives in trees and learned to crack bullwhips, fire slingshots, and hurl axes and hand-fashioned spears. We swam considerable distances behind the rowboat, stayed underwater as long as we could, and met any other challenge that showed prowess or cunning. A.J. was especially fond of tug-of-war, so we played that game often. Another favorite was capture the flag. One jet-black night I was all alone, creeping through deep grass in a distant meadow, on the point of crossing into enemy territory, and a pheasant took flight from the high grass directly in front of me. I felt as if my heart would fly out of my breast. I continued to shudder long after I had recognized the source of my terror.

Scouting also meant unforgettable mischief. Once I was strongly shocked by an electric fence that two of my friends dared me to touch. Another time, in a mood, I used my sling-shot and some metal balls or marbles to shoot at a handful of cows mired in muck along the riverbank until they stampeded. I was afraid that one of them might break her leg in the desperate ascent up the sloping riverbank.

I've never forgotten my own initiation to Troop 118. I and my fellow inductees were made to suck the end of a rope, being told it was a snake's tail. We had to jump to the ground from "eight feet in the air" (when in fact I was standing on a bench mere inches off the ground), and to brave an arduous snake walk (a succession of nasty pranks by older scouts). At the culmination of the snake walk, I fought as I never had fought in my life when the older scouts, along with A.J., unsuccessfully tried to tie me to a tombstone in a remote country cemetery.

Memorable too were the tests that measured our characters and unique physical traits. I chickened out of a fight with Mike Street, the strongest of us all, when he called me a "Dago." He was standing at the boat landing, and I was standing on the high bank above. It was a long way down to the landing, and I didn't believe I had a chance against the short, barrel-chested Mike Street, who at twelve or thirteen pressed 160 pounds the first time he lifted weights.

"Fluid-Drive Schroeder" consistently won our pissing contests. We would stand in a line, with penises out, lay out a log and keep moving it back from where we stood to find out who was the longest pisser of all. Invariably, it was "Fluid-Drive Schroeder," whose tall body and matching penis emitted a great arching stream that cleared the log—and helped extinguish the sparks of many a campfire as well.

At camp we boys practiced being men. There was an order of strength in which I fit toward the top, but I was nowhere near as strong as Mike. Fishing and hunting skills also produced a hierarchy, at whose apex stood Mike along with Doug Rahn. Doug hunted with his dad, and Mike had in his basement his own actual den, a converted coal bin in which he kept rocks, birds' nests, artificial flies and lures, a sharp hunting knife with a holster, a real deer skull, and many copies of

Field and Stream, which opened doors to great adventures in the wild.

Ron stood closer to Mike and Doug in woods skill and lore than I did. Although I bought equipment—a bow, a hunting knife, a fishing pole—I lacked any grace with them. I aimed my bow poorly. I spent my time fishing, unraveling backlashes, and retrieving my lures from snags and trees. On one squirrel hunting escapade, I slipped on the ice and broke all the arrows in my quiver. I went home alone, ashamed and angry. Remembering that I never was much good on expeditions, I feared bad luck on the operation ahead.

Ron and I quit scouts at the same time for the same reason. We had started caddying at the Country Club of Detroit in nearby Grosse Pointe Farms. Weekly scouting meetings in the grade school kindergarten room no longer seemed fun. A.J. didn't want me to leave, but Ron and I had made up our minds—or perhaps, in truth, Ron had made up his mind for both of us. Ron, one of A.J.'s life scouts, and I, a newly initiated member of the Order of the Arrow, left Troop 118.

For our two years before high school, Ron and I were glued together by caddying. We went to and from the course together, hung together at the caddie house, and spent our evenings together. We wore the same style of clothes, were musically initiated by Bill Hailey's Comets, and spent a lot of time just being together. We lit cigarettes off each other and shared drags. When we had only one match left, Ron could be counted on to get his lit. He had a knack for cupping his hand

and lighting his cigarette by facing into the wind. One time his mother passed by in a car while Ron was lighting a cigarette. He quickly put his hand in his pocket so she wouldn't see him smoking, but inadvertently set the lining of his brand-new leather aviator's jacket on fire. Discovering he was on fire, Ron took his coat off and jumped up and down on it. No sooner had he stopped jumping than he started nervously guessing what would happen when his mother and father found out.

We usually hitchhiked to the golf course. We idled away our time between loops, often went out together on the same round, and gossiped about the same players. We had no sympathy for the short old men with crooked, skinny legs who wore short pants. We liked the young women with big breasts and swaying rears, whom the boldest caddies followed with lurid gestures. We eavesdropped on the conversations of young men who hit the ball a long way, gambled, and indiscreetly joked about their manly escapades. We held court over members' tips. Ron especially liked the members who said witty things. He would repeat phrases he'd heard for days on end, highlighting them with his infectious laughter.

The caddie house was a second home for Ron and me. Together we sneaked off to the old hole—an abandoned hole from a course layout—to practice. Occasionally we abandoned the course altogether and went out to nearby Lake St. Claire to sneak a swim at the yachting club. We competed with each other at golf, especially on the putting green. Ron caddied for me the year I won the club's caddie championship. As a team we sized up my putts together, I stroked the ball, and into the cup it went. I got six or seven birdies in the twenty-eight holes it took me to win the thirty-six-hole match.

We often stayed at the course putting until the sun went down. On those nights, we took the bus home to his place and then set off for the nearby ice cream parlor, where a waitress named Eunice awakened our dawning sexual interest. Eunice was stunningly beautiful and several years older than us. We repeatedly tried to give her the largest tip she'd ever gotten. We paid double the price for our banana splits and hoped that our beloved doe-eyed and sharp-breasted Eunice would look affectionately at us.

One morning while we were waiting for a bus to the course, Ron offered me an "I Like Ike" cigarette. I accepted. After having quit for three months, I was hooked again. I never quite forgave him for that. And this vicious twenty-five-year habit and my damaged heart condition was something else to lay at the Republican Party's doorstep.

On overnights at Ron's house we slept in the basement in an unfinished room he shared with his younger brother, Joe. Next to the room stood the household's great coal furnace. Ron was its keeper, the Hephaestus of this fire. He fed its great stoker, poked the dark smoldering cinders, and reached into this crucible with great tongs, withdrawing the giant clinkers, placing them in large metal buckets that he carried outside once they cooled. My father had converted our house to gas several years before. He turned our coal bin into a storage closet, set up a work bench in the newly freed space, and put a wall around the old furnace area, creating a tool room. Ron's basement was more elemental than ours. In his basement, soot and dust pervaded my lungs, and I was in awe of the fiery furnace. It promised the same sort of dreadful transformation as the operating table that lay in wait for me.

The roughness of Ron's basement corresponded to the undecorated upstairs. His home contained just the essentials. The minimal furniture in the kitchen, front room, and dining room was old; there were no drapes or doilies, no pictures on the walls, no collections of knickknacks or photographs on any of the shelves. The house lacked the touch of an involved housewife. I was too young to conclude anything from this, but I couldn't help perceiving the difference between his home and mine, with its freshly painted walls, carpeted floors, draped windows, bountiful doilies, crystal chandelier, china closet, and my mother's teacup collection.

Ron's handsome red-haired mother sold things and had a temper. His father, a heavy man who suffered from fits of gout, which drove him to using a cane, occasionally strummed a few bars on his Jew's harp for us. He told stories of his days down south in Georgia, which Ron cherished. Once in a while, to Ron's delight, his father took to singing "Beat Your Feet on the Mississippi Mud." I knew his father often stopped at a bar before he came home from work, and Ron had to go and fetch him home more than once. The hints were there, but I was young and had no experience with which to conjecture how much alcohol ravaged Ron's family. Later, when he and I were no longer the closest of friends, his mother died a long and nasty death from cancer, after having burned herself in bed.

These pre-high school years were golden years for me. My home was stable. I was confident that I was loved. I had not yet encountered failure in high school or on the golf course. And I had not yet determined that girls were creatures I could please or who could please me. They were as mysterious to me as the pimples that had sprung up on my forehead.

Ron was much better with the girls than I was. He enjoyed being with them. He enjoyed joking and teasing in their company. He knew how to flirt with them, and he paid attention to his hair, dress, and shoes. He used deodorant as well as aftershave lotion, even though he didn't have a beard. He also had a better idea of what girls' bodies and his pleasures were about. I knew little, other than that ejaculation was a shudderingly pleasant event, even though the church left no doubt in my mind that it was wrong.

Until our seventh-grade graduation party at Catherine De Luca's, I had no notion of what sex was. That night a tall, thin, German girl with braces French kissed me and everyone else she could set her large, open mouth on. In the small, musty basement, girls and boys who had sat next to each other in class for seven years for the first time kissed and pushed their irregularly shaped bodies up against one another. Upstairs, right next to the cake, sat the host's jaundiced grandfather. A small, old, yellow man, he couldn't speak, had long fingernails, and smelt powerfully of urine. The big creamy cake next to him wasn't very tasty that day. I felt vaguely ashamed that a person could smell so foul and be in such a condition, and I was confused that girls could kiss so hard and enthusiastically.

Ron had several girlfriends even before he went to high school, whereas in my entire freshman year I had only one date. Although it involved a long walk to and from her house and a bus trip to and from a football game, it yielded only a handful of clumsy sentences framed by awkward silences. She didn't tell or ask me anything, and I failed to interest her in golf. Her refusal to kiss me goodnight crowned a wasted night, and boded ill for the future of my body-to-body and heart-to-heart relationships with the opposite sex.

If I did badly with girls, I did worse in school. In the ninth grade I flunked algebra. I barely got through Spanish with a D. I did the same in biology. My sophomore year was a repeat performance, except that I withdrew from geometry before I failed it. (My mother kept all my report cards to remind me never to be too hard on my own children.) By the second half of my sophomore year, I was moved into the business curriculum. It was clear that I wasn't good at anything in school, except possibly the social sciences and history.

Because Ron and I were at different high schools—Ron at Southeastern and I at Denby—we saw each other less and less. Even in summers we saw less of each other as my interest in golf exceeded his and my hours at the driving range kept me at the course until late every night. He made new friends at Southeastern while I became more and more solitary. Then, for no clear reason that I could ever figure out, I emerged during the last half of my junior year as a socialite. I became a member of the most popular high school fraternity and was elected to class office. I was captain of the high school golf team that won the city competition and a state letter, and I switched to college preparatory courses, determined to get good grades. My pimples disappeared—as my mom said they would—and I dressed well. I wore white bucks, had a tan suede jacket, and sported a letter sweater.

During our junior and senior years Ron and I met occasionally at golf tournaments that pitted Southeastern against Denby. But we lived in different worlds. We were superficially reunited at the University of Michigan when he arrived to live at the Evans Scholars House a year after I did.

꿍

I arrived early at the bar to meet Ron. I was anxious to talk about events that had happened forty years before, those singular, irreplaceable times when we were boys together. As my bypass stood in the way of my future, it made me hunger for the past. Waiting for Ron was like waiting for so many unnamed but needed memories. Only a friend could supply the memories that would allow me to say my farewell to my past and myself. Expectation swelled as my wait extended. I felt as if Ron and I had just been with each other a few days before, as if I were waiting for him to finish his caddying loop so we could set out for the ice cream parlor and green-eyed Eunice.

Ron showed up late, as he often used to, and arrived with a small entourage: his wife, Mimi, and a couple of his law interns. Ron always liked to have a small group around him. My fear that they would block our road to the past quickly vanished. Ron and I paired off as Mimi and the interns started a conversation among themselves.

I was struck by how vital Ron appeared. His complexion was good; his eyes were keen, steady, and bright. I was not surprised when he told me that he had recently won a bike race and that he was still able to out-ride his sons, who were in their late teens. His lake place up north supported his health regimen.

Over the years Ron had worked for a law firm, specializing in union contracts. His politics, which took its full form in the first years of his marriage, remained liberal Democratic. He had remained loyal to "the teams without uniforms," the kind of team we had played for under the captaincy of Donnie Sam. By choice, he lived in the city in a mixed neighborhood.

I let Ron know that I shared his views on unionism, war protest, and social justice. With a keen rudder, I steered clear of issues like abortion and affirmative action. I didn't want to risk mixing reminiscence with ideology. And I wanted to assure him, even though I doubted that I could, that I was not the zealot I had been during my junior and senior years at the university, when I had talked of little else other than Catholicism.

Ron asked about my family, especially my mother, who had always liked him. And I asked about his family. I wanted to know how his three brothers had fared. Since I had first read Dostoevsky's *The Brothers Karamazov,* Ron and his brothers had reminded me of those brothers. Ron talked openly about his family. His older brother, Tom, had committed suicide many years before. A mixture of earnestness, passion, and sensuality, Tom had never quite found his way in work or marriage. His second brother, Gene, was Tom's antithesis. Gene had disciplined himself to succeed but in the process had, it seemed to Ron, crushed a part of the emotional life within him. He became a distinguished eye surgeon, but couldn't help Ron cope with their parents or face Tom's suicide. Ron himself had sought a difficult and delicate balance between Tom's sensuality and Gene's self-discipline, between his father's jovial corporeality and his mother's intense psychology. Ron's youngest brother, Joe, seemed the least ambitious and complex of the four. Gentle and kind, he was the family Alyosha.

Although I was disappointed in Ron's memories of our country club days, having expected them to be more detailed and sensual, they nevertheless contained essential elements of the past. Our conversation accomplished what I most wanted—it made distant childhood days present. We taunted A.J. at camp, played ball for Donnie Sam, sneaked into the yacht club, and putted until it was dark. I had my farewell party.

As we rose to say good-bye, I was filled with gratitude for a past that had been awakened in me. I didn't mention my pending open-heart surgery to Ron. I didn't want to spoil memories of a time when our senses were fresh with the world's imprint, when our bodies and minds were one, and when we—scouts and caddies—could walk on and on without tiring.

There were other reasons why I didn't make my bypass a subject for conversation. I had determined on some level where choice really doesn't count to take on this operation tight-lipped. It was my World War II, my private battle. Furthermore, talk of my pending bypass made me vulnerable to pity.

Besides, it was just bad form to not see a person for decades and then talk about the possibility of your death. And what could Ron have said? What could I have said? I would either falsely dismiss it as a trifle or it would dominate everything else. One way or another, I realized, this matter of heart would dominate all others. It was much better to talk of times when spirit and flesh were fresh, when life came in rich, juicy bits, and to hear that Ron—one of the better bicycle riders of our gang—could still out-race his sons.

First Pains

The next morning I drove out to the Country Club of Detroit, in Grosse Pointe Farms, where forty-five years before, as a boy of twelve, I started to caddie and where I received my first education in heartbreak.

John Standish, club member, bank president, and supporter of a scholarship program for caddies, had invited me to have lunch with him at the club. I had written to him to request a visit in order to do some research on a book I was writing on golf. On the way there I remembered our Sunday family drives out to Grosse Pointe to see the estates that fronted Lake Saint Claire. We would pass the mansions with "oohs" whose volume and emphasis measured each estate's size and opulence. We always culminated our tour at Ford's estate. My family considered it the greatest mansion of all, first because it belonged to the Fords, and second because it was as immense as any home we could imagine, hidden behind a small wood and a stone wall anchored by a gatehouse that was larger than any house in our neighborhood.

As a caddie at the country club I learned about the privileges of class. Uniformed black men, with cheery "Yes, sirs," manned the locker room, foyer, bar and grill, and half-way house. Italians manned the pro shop and the caddie house, while predominantly working- and lower-middle-class kids filled out the ranks of caddies. We carried bags for members named Lord and Highby. Their manners, toys, and games, which included debutante parties, sports cars, and polo, were different from those of the people of my neighborhood.

It was this country club introduction to class differences that formed my golfing sympathies for players who, like myself, came off the public courses and out of the caddie shacks and pro shops rather than from country clubs and universities. It also played a part in my becoming a self-declared socialist as a senior in high school. My conversion was aided by reading John Steinbeck's *In Dubious Battle*.

As I entered the secluded drive that led into the country club, I felt I had re-entered my youth. The three-story, English country-estate clubhouse with its high, gabled, black slate roof had not been altered a bit, and it seemed to command the unchanging world that surrounded it. It would remain whether I did or not. It was one of those places that outlasted people and generations.

Inside the clubhouse, an air of permanence clung to the stone walls and high wood ceilings. On one wall I saw framed the *Sports Illustrated* article that featured Arnold Palmer and Robert Sweeny's duel to win the 1954 National Amateur at our course. At the center of the article was a photograph of my friend, Ron Helveston. With his hand on his hip and his elbow out, turned halfway between his player and the green, Ron appeared absorbed by Sweeny's dilemma of trying to recover from a seriously pushed tee shot on the thirty-sixth and final hole of the match. A gigantic elm stood directly along the line of his approach to the distant and highly trapped and elevated eighteenth green, which, surrounded by trees in the back, sat below the long stone clubhouse porch.

The '54 Amateur was the biggest golfing event in the club's history and in my life as a caddie. Disappointingly, I had gotten the bag of a stocky, pock-marked Los Angeles restauranteur in his late thirties or early forties. He had none of the excitement of the wild-hitting Bill-Jo Patton, the flash and toughness of the emerging young Arnold Palmer, or the elegance of the silver-haired aristocratic Sweeny. Yet my man followed a first-day bye with a brilliant round. He closed his opponent on the fourteenth hole on his way toward a course record round. That day I clubbed him perfectly and lined up his putts flawlessly. The next day things went badly. On the eleventh hole, I insisted he hit an eight rather than a nine, which he wanted to play. He hit the ball over the green and into the back rough. By the sixteenth hole he was done for. I felt I had failed him. He gave me a two-dollar tip for each round, which included a practice round, for twenty or thirty dollars in all. My friend Ron received five hundred dollars from Sweeny.

I remembered, as I sat drinking a beer waiting for Mr. Standish, who had been delayed, how I once bungled a tip from Henry Ford II, who was the best tipper at the club. On the second hole, a long par-four that was reachable by very few players, Mr. Ford saw players on the green ahead and, after what was a very good drive for him, asked me whether he could get home. I replied, "Not in one." He showed such delight in my answer that I concluded he wanted a comic for a caddie. On the fourth hole, he drove his ball wickedly into the woods on the right. Blocked from any possible approach to the green, he asked what he should do. I replied, repeating an old golf joke, "Pray." Mr. Ford didn't find my remark at all funny. He refused to talk to me during the rest of the round. My tip of fifty cents for eighteen from Mr. Ford was the all-time caddie-house low.

I remembered caddying for Mr. Stroh of Stroh's Brewery one day. Stroh sliced his short drive into the deep, leaf-covered rough of the par-five third. As I was looking for his ball, he told me he had found it, and before I could say anything he swung. Stroh was nearly blind and looked like he carried a barrel of his brew in his protruding stomach. I looked up and realized he had mistakenly addressed and hit a mushroom. When he asked me where his shot had gone, I was forced to reply, "Sir, you struck a mushroom, sir." He replied, "Oh!" and continued to look for his ball, as if hitting mushrooms was nothing out of the ordinary.

Still waiting for Standish, I walked out on to the porch and surveyed the course, which for a time I had known as well as any caddie knows a course. My thoughts turned to how I had invested the passions of my youth in golf only to discover that life does not grant what one most wants and works for. Failures break hearts.

⚬—⫻—⚬

As a boy, I couldn't be happier than when I set out on my bike on the two-mile ride to Chandler Park, the east side's public golf course, with a bag of rattling clubs on my shoulder. I was at home on what now seems a pinched parcel of green, bordered by a public park along one side and sliced tangentially along the other by I-94, the immense throughway that paved over my boyhood home and dissected the heart of my neighborhood my junior year in high school.

At Chandler Park I worked my own magic, suffered my own errors, and harvested the fruits of my own efforts. Golf's pleasures were vivid and immediate, so sharply different from school's drudgery. Golf was my craft. I knew its rules far better than I knew the rules of mathematics, natural science, English, and Spanish.

The game was about me. It was about my aim, my swing, the flight of my ball, and my final score. I was as absorbed with golf as I was with myself. In fact, the absorption was in large part one and the same. Golf was my tie to self, to society, to life; it was my way of being serious, responsible, and hopeful. When I caddied, I played the member's round in my mind as if it were my own, all the while keeping an eye peeled for a stray ball or two for my late evening practice or play. On the tee, waiting for the members to finish putting, I'd pick up a club, test its heft and lie, and give it a swing. The swing, a pleasure in itself, swished across space and time, joining hand and body in one smooth flow.

On the course I was free. I was a boy among boys, a true equal among competing equals. We bet, cursed, smoked, and played as long as daylight and weather permitted. Our legs were tireless; our matches were keen. We did not hesitate to challenge the best players on the course. I remember once in a skins game (in which the lowest score on a hole wins) with two older men, Ron purposely missed a four-footer so I could make a three-footer in order to take both men's money with a winning birdie 3. I felt more proud about making that putt than I felt guilty about cheating them out of their money.

I played out my desire to be a professional golfer on two entirely different courses. The first was the short, hard, bush- and tree-lined Chandler Park. While the holes were laid out mechanically back and forth and up and down, the small greens, tight fairways, and a few treacherous traps gave the course a degree of difficulty. When the wind was up, success required a range of shots, especially bump-and-run shots.

In contrast, the Country Club of Detroit—which measured my highest aspirations—was a true championship course. Its long-manicured tees, molded fairways traversed by bunkers, deep roughs, and elevated and flawless greens made it a test at all times, especially since it had been redesigned by one of golf's great architects, Robert Trent Jones, for the 1954 National Amateur. Shots there had to fly long and high and had to be on target. Each nine had a couple of truly difficult par fours. If you couldn't play out of every kind of sand trap, you couldn't play there. I never tread on the country club course without thinking, if I am not good here, I will never be a worthy golfer.

Like every decent player, I had my wonderful moments in

the game. In those moments I would be lifted out of my ordinary play. I would beat someone better than myself, win a little money, make a truly smart or clever shot, or make a lovely hole-in-one. I would see a shot in my mind, swing, and the shot I had visualized would fly effortlessly through the air to its target as if commanded by a higher force.

In the final round of the caddie championship, I enjoyed the pleasure of near perfect putting. I lined up my putts, aimed, and then struck the ball. It rolled as if it had eyes right into the cup. I made seven birdies in the thirty or fewer holes it took me to win. That day I was crowned caddie champion and truly felt like a master of the game. I believed I could make my living golfing.

On most days, however, the course defeated me. Like a mountain, it repelled my strongest ascents, made once a week on caddie's day. Even when I was off it, it loomed over me with the single imposing thought that I could never shoot par on it and, thus, I would never be a professional golfer.

Painful days on the golf course introduced me, round by round, to dark corners of my mind I had never known. I had fallen in love with the game. I had taken its terrible allurement of perfection to heart: I would command my body and propel the ball through space with perfection. I would thread my shots as carefully through the course as I hoped surgeons would snip and sew segments of a breast artery and a leg vein to my heart. Invariably, my play disappointed. I never met the exacting standards I set or satisfied the dreams I cultivated. I was young and in love with the game, though, so at first I rebounded quickly from bad rounds. I needed only a day or two of recuperation and with a few swishes of my driver I again was filled with golfing hopes. I was sure that I would arise from the ranks of caddies to the lofty realm of professional golfers, as had Sarazen, Hogan, Snead, and Nelson.

As my family members dedicated their energies to make a living in the factories of Detroit, so I dedicated myself to perfecting my golf game. When I wasn't out at a course, I swung and chipped in the backyard. When I was at the course, I went out back of the caddie house between loops and chipped from tree to tree, or went down to the old hole and practiced midirons. I never missed playing on caddie's day, which was always on Monday morning. I would start close to sunrise and play among the sprinklers. Once in a while, caddie master Caesar Raimondi let Ron and me play a late nine after work. We often finished our round putting in the moonlight.

I was always among the first to open the golf season at Chandler Park. One year I played between mounds of melting snow and on half-frozen fairways and greens. At school I practiced gripping my pencils as if they were clubs and played imaginary rounds as my teachers droned on and on. My obsession with mastery of the game reached a crescendo during my junior year when I began to run the club's driving range. There I would hit balls hour after hour. I learned to hit long, short, high, and low shots, fades and draws, and shots from different lies, all of which were required to master what I argued (confidently and tediously) was surely the world's most intriguing and complex sport.

On the range I had days of ecstasy. My swing found a natural tempo and rhythm. I could hit any shot I wanted to. At those times I was fooled into believing that I had reached a new plateau, and I was on my way to being a professional. But the range also offered its share of pain. With all the balls I wanted to hit, I was like a glutton before too much food. I would practice until the calluses on my hands split and bled—and still I would hit more balls. The better I hit my shots, the better I expected to hit them. It was as if the closer I came to my goal, the further it receded. Most painful was that a good practice session frequently preceded terrible play. I would stumble off the course feeling betrayed and nauseated. Dark emotions of bitter defeat and self-disgust swirled within me.

At times I felt as if I had two swings, one for the driving range and another for the course. Sometimes I even felt that what I did on the range didn't matter. A couple of times I quit playing for a week only to return to the game to repeat the cycle of hope, desperation, and despair. I was too proud to acknowledge that a game could get me so down. Like a tormented lover, I couldn't be with or away from the person I loved. And golf had such a fickle heart.

Golf so punished me that it led to my first conscious experiments with philosophy. Believing I must make it to the pros by age eighteen or not at all, and running out of faith that practice would make a difference, I tried to improve my game by changing my attitude. First I tried Dale Carnegie's fashionable "power of positive thinking": If I expected good shots, I'd hit good shots. When this forced optimism quickly failed, I substituted a thoroughgoing pessimism. I would expect the worst in hopes of being surprised by the good. Unfortunately, I immediately got the terrible results I anticipated. I abandoned my willed fatalism the very first day I experimented with it.

No single humiliation was as great as losing the caddie championship in my senior year. I played badly and lost to a caddie a year my junior whose last name was D'Amato. I was losing my heart for the game.

Golf was a cruel friend. It lifted me up only to drive me down. I came to understand with Buddha-like enlightenment that golf's pleasures chained me to its painful illusions. I voiced my emerging adult pessimism with the first lines of poetry I ever wrote:

Some men strive
To discover life a meaningless hive.
While others crave
To find life a bottomless grave.

I started to substitute golf's glory with pride in my ability to think. I took philosophy to heart. If I could not defeat golf on the course, I would encompass it by my understanding. A mere boy, I determined in my heart that I would meet life with clear thought even if that included a willingness to concede defeat in having what I most wanted. Forty years ago, golf taught me the attitude I adopted toward my forthcoming bypass: I would lie down and accept what the skills of others, luck, and grace yielded.

One day, in the late summer just before I started my junior year of high school, golf suddenly became secondary to me because of a decision I still can't fathom. For no explainable reason, on my way out of the milk depot, where I had gone to buy a gallon of milk, I realized with the full force of consciousness that I would go to college. As a consequence of what might be considered a kind of conversion, I immediately jumped from being a D+ to an A student. Even though I won several high school golf matches and tournaments, captained a city championship team, and finished eighth out of more than three hundred young regional golfers (finishing the last eighteen with a 72), the game gave way in my life to reading and a new-found high school popularity that catapulted me into the position of senior class officer.

Golf now became only something I played. I would not spend my whole life desiring such a fickle mistress. Instead, I would pursue studies that rewarded steady effort and whose primary instruments, pencils, had erasers. Golf's hold over me was completely broken when I was awarded a four-year Standish-Evans caddie scholarship for tuition and room at the University of Michigan. Golf had paid off after all. My father, who had never held a golf club in his hands, was proud. His son was doing what he would have done if he had had the chance. I was the first of my entire family to go to the university—and the University of Michigan at that! My novitiate on the links was finished. My place in the garden of knowledge had yet to be determined.

⁕

John Standish and I spent our lunch together reminiscing. We spoke of old members, changes in the club and the game, and the '54 Amateur. He gave me a brief history of the country club and invited me back to play sometime. I was grateful. Of course, I never mentioned that I had also come to say a provisional good-bye to the course and the part of my youth it represented.

I stopped at the caddie shack before leaving. In place of the short, stocky, and powerful Caesar who had run the shack in my day I found a tall, quiet, gentle young man who referred to himself as a "golf resource manager." He furnished members with golf carts, which to a large degree had replaced the caddies. Inside the caddie shed I saw further evidence of the caddie's declining importance. The 25-by-15 foot room had not been painted for a long time. On the cement floor sat the same long, blond-slat benches (taken from the club's bowling alley) on which I had sat four decades earlier. On those benches we had killed time waiting for a loop by talking, playing cards, catching flies, drinking pop, and eating Twinkies. The benches on one side of the shed had been shortened to make room for three large video games. The video games expressed an instancy foreign to the long, slow rhythms of walking, sitting, and talking that had defined my boyhood. They were companions of the computers that fly self-directing missiles—the type that surgically pulverized Iraq—and the lasers that were experimentally being used to open blocked arteries.

The back door of the shed was blocked. The caddies had lost access to the space behind the shed and the pro shop where, between loops, we had spent our idle time. They could no longer sit in the shade of the porch, which faced the basketball court, nor could they go beyond the court out into the caddie's yard, an L-shaped area of grass and sand under the canopy of small scotch pines where we had passed whole days practicing chip shots, playing horseshoes, and wise-cracking.

Caddies now also could not walk over to the driving range, where they might pick up a few tips from one of the assistant pros or pocket a sly ball or two for playing a match at the old hole. The old hole itself no longer existed. Years ago, it had been gobbled up to create a new three-hole executive course.

The caddies' place in the game had been eclipsed—they were a dying breed. Former caddies once had dominated the ranks of professional golf, from the era of Quimet and Sarazen through the age of Hogan and Nelson. Now they no longer supplied players for the game. Caddies have gone the way of many old breeds, like household servants, chimney sweeps, and my peasant grandparents from Sicily.

As I drove out of the lot, I remembered once reading in Herbert Warren Wind's *The Story of American Golf* that in the building of one of America's first great courses, William Vanderbilt (son of American railway magnate Cornelius Vanderbilt) and Scottish pro Willie Dunn transformed four thousand acres along Great Peconic Bay into a twelve-hole golf course using a crew of 150 men from the nearby Shinnecock Indian reservation. These men cleared the fairways, removed blueberry bushes from the rough, and—in a display of how civilizations ravage the heritage of those that precede them—"utilized the Indian burial mounds as obstacles before the greens or made them into sand traps."

Perhaps my family was like the Shinnecock Indians. We were drawn to Detroit to make the nation's cars. Then we made its tanks and planes during the Second World War. We built our life around this new industrial order and this order over time consumed its own, as all capitalist systems do. In any case, by virtue of being a caddie and a son of industrial workers, I was numbered among the living dead. Life was passing me by. I prognosticated a time when my grandchildren would grasp the lives of those who constructed the pyramids of Egypt as easily as they would understand me and their great grandparents, who worked for Henry Ford and his kind.

Chrysalis

I spent an evening and last day of my three-day trip to Michigan in Ann Arbor. I went there to visit Professor Stephen Tonsor, my first intellectual mentor. During my four years at the University of Michigan, from 1956 to 1960, I felt I was drowning and Tonsor's ideas offered the first traces of solid land.

In one sense Tonsor (whose name implies clipping, shearing, etc.) was my first heart surgeon. His ideas allowed me to transfuse my heart with fresh blood. Thanks to him and his authentication of the religious view of human experience, I no longer believed that my heart must be divided forever between my thoughts and feelings. What I inherited was credible; faith was legitimate; hope was possible. To see Tonsor on the eve of my bypass, even if I did not whisper a single word about it to him, was a worthy pilgrimage — an act of homage to the Virgil who helped lead me through and beyond the Inferno of self-consciousness into which I had fallen.

I had a theory about the origin of the terrible self-consciousness that settled upon me as soon as I arrived at the university. I was from the working classes, the only one in the family who ever went to college. By going to college, I separated myself from my family and what traditions we had. I made myself into a head without a body.

My mother had a simpler explanation, one she claimed the parish priest had given her: "Your son will lose his faith if he goes to the University of Michigan." When she was in a bad mood about my being single and not going to church, she attacked the books I read and the friends I kept. She particularly focused on my high school English teacher, Mr. Lux, who had us read good literature—even pieces from *The New Yorker*—and once revealed to a few of us students that he was an atheist.

In any case, she was right about me taking ideas too seriously. I became a socialist upon reading Steinbeck as a junior in high school. A senior paper on H. L. Mencken made me a free-wheeling critic of society. I was against everything and anything that was part of what I perceived to be dull middle-class society.

Overlooking a short period in my senior year when I got straight A's in chemistry and intended to become a metallurgical engineer, I had no respect for technology. I didn't note significant advances in medicine, and I scorned the first Russian sputnik as an extension of the arms race into the heavens.

Jazz, brooding poetry, dark Russian novels, and all things Spanish—especially bull fighting, flamenco music, and Hemingway novels—won my heart. I embraced a counterculture whose first target was middle-class suburban life. I took it to be the antithesis of a meaningful existence. I started a long poem titled "White Crane" in which I spoke about a "world flying kites into sky-written skies / turning primitive pots in contemporary buildings / waiting for a brown apocalypse." I shared my generation's confusion over whether the world would end in nuclear conflagration or simply evaporate amid well-tended lawns and air-conditioning.

With my golf clubs and skates at the back of my closet, my only pleasures were long walks and late-night conversations. They were my heart's university of budding feelings and thoughts. Dave Lyon taught me about jazz, chess, and contemporary literature and art, until he flunked out of the university playing billiards. Many nights I walked around with another high school friend, Richard Beekman. Though he planned to be a nuclear physicist, he joined my fear of emasculation in the suburbs. One night we drank some cheap wine and shared a vow never to push a lawn mower in the suburbs and to travel to the old country to seek out a traditional wife.

My friendships with fellow Evans Scholars Ron Helveston, Jew Jerry Char, and Mexican Renato Gonzalez also led me against the grain. While living in the scholarship home, we stood against the conformities that went with our brothers' effort to transform us lower-class kids into a bright and shining fraternity. We resisted joining their intramural sports teams (although I played a little handball), singing in their choirs, and serenading our Greek sisters. They cajoled us about our unkempt appearance and took insult when one of us failed to greet a recently pinned sister. They levied fines to enforce behavior. I was once fined ten dollars for not going to the house's spring ball. At one meeting, my first experiment in public speaking, I told them they were barnacles stuck on the fraternity ship, and I didn't care which horizon they sailed over. They soon found a way to put me, Char, Helveston, and others who didn't have "house spirit" out into the recently acquired house annex.

I cultivated a rebelliousness that was instinctive. I didn't take well to forced popularity. I considered a declaration that studying engineering or business was tantamount to a confession of dullness and betrayal of spirit. I judged other disciplines and career ambitions equally sharply, but none as mercilessly as psychology, which I judged to be a hoax: There could be no science of mind. Its self-evident experiments and always banal and badly written conclusions proved it. After just a few weeks of classes of introductory psychology, I told the teacher that I wouldn't learn anything in her class. She graciously replied that I should just show up for the final examination, which I did. I got a B after one night's study.

My romance with formal philosophy, which should have been the romance of my life, ended the very day I set out to get information on becoming a philosophy major. I entered the basement of Angell Hall looking for a philosophy teacher, hearing the voices of my family shouting in my ear: "How is a kid from Ithaca going to make a living in Athens talking?" I didn't find a counselor. (I even remember passing the darkened office of the well-known logician Irving Copi.) Just before leaving Angell Hall, I wandered into a small room. At the back, in front of a large portable chalkboard, stood two graduate students. They were pondering row upon row of complex formulae. I asked them what they were doing. They said they were working on a truth equation. St. Paul wasn't knocked off his horse any more quickly. In one blinding instant, I knew I wasn't going be a philosopher if truth required facility with the advanced algebra whose rudimentary beginnings I failed as a freshman in high school.

I had entered Angell Hall feeling like a bird honing homeward after a long and errant career flight. I left it sensing I had been plucked of every last feather—like a rum-dumb Icarus, who had fallen to ground before he had even taken flight.

Shortly after entering college, I shed my romance with being a labor lawyer and helping Marlon Brando's brother run the docks in the film *On the Waterfront*. Those ambitions went down the drain at the fraternity where I washed dishes with two law students. One seemed truly mentally disorganized. Gaunt, with a shadow of a beard, he always looked like he had just tumbled out of bed. The second was his opposite: a short, roly-poly fellow who beamed with good cheer. Together they convinced me that the study of law must be for odd and superficial people. Furthermore, seven years of university constituted too long an interval before getting on with one's life.

After abandoning English because I couldn't write, there was nothing left for me but history. So I became a history major—and bowing to a working-class man's need to earn a living, I sought a secondary teacher's certificate. I arrived at the school of education filled with the standing liberal arts prejudices against education. These prejudices were quickly confirmed by what I experienced. In one course, we were required to prepare a bulletin board (an assignment my mom did for me). In a history of education course, I got another B with a single night's study.

My dislike of psychology and education came together in educational psychology. One day our instructor concluded his hour-long lecture with the argument that the contemporary explanation of the brain as a chemical-electrical matter of neurons and synapses is the best account we have of human thought. He completed his argument with the illogical statement that what he said was true because it couldn't be disproved. I immediately asked him if the angel playing the harpsichord during his lecture had disturbed him. I hastened to explain that he couldn't disprove that a celestial musician had not accompanied his lecture.

A few days later, after class, I accompanied him to his office. Partly out of curiosity, and partly hoping to restore amicable relations, I asked him what his doctoral dissertation topic was. When he replied, "learning machines," I responded, "If I had a child who didn't break the machines, I would break him." He dubbed me "a rebel without a cause," a description I took—not having seen the James Dean movie of that name— as a compliment.

For my first three years at the university, I was alone and angry. I was angry—if in retrospect I try to offer reasons—

because the city of Detroit ran a giant interstate expressway over my house and through my neighborhood, casting us out into the sterile suburbs of East Detroit. I was angry, though not conscious of it, because my family had been on an uninterrupted migration for the past hundred years, forcing us to constantly adjust our minds and ways to those of strangers. I also was angry because my generation had no war to fight, as my uncles had. We just had goods — televisions, cars, record players, and other things to enjoy. But I was indifferent to, and even disdained, what others strove for.

There was a simpler explanation for my anger, one that would have pleased the educational psychologists. I simply didn't fit in. I didn't quite know how to be around others. I was an only child, and I lacked skills siblings acquire of how to fight and forgive. Also, I had no sisters by which to take intimate measure of what girls were made of. At the university I was out of my class and culture. While I knew how to be ingratiating and was not easily intimidated, I was clumsy in the presence of those who were rich, educated, and mannered. The mere display of a few upper-class mannerisms and I tended to revert to a subservient caddie. Education, which filled me with aspirations, also made me feel inferior in countless ways, and contemporary dreams of success had not yet grafted me to society's skin.

As I drove to Ann Arbor, I was struck by how often in life I ended up alone, things always seeming to turn on the matter of this head versus that world. Trying to piece things together, to impose an order on them, has always been my compelling duty and my neurotic way. Now I faced my forthcoming bypass almost in the comfort of my own solitude, while in university days insecurity, anxiety, and dreams filled my loneliness.

That loneliness was intensified by my episodic relationships with women. I liked talking to them about serious things, and I enjoyed hugging and kissing them. But of what lay beyond I had neither a clear biological idea nor even a commonplace grasp. I had no idea how one chose a woman and abided with her. I only knew that one day you liked someone, then you got serious, then you got married. You went to bed together and had as much sex as you desired, and so produced the family that your parents wanted you to have. Beyond that, I was ignorant of how flesh and feeling fit together in friendship and marriage.

By dating I sought to satiate a hunger I didn't understand. It always resulted in more pain and confusion than pleasure and companionship. However many dates I had, the icy grip of self-consciousness never weakened its hold on my mind.

I gave up on the first girl I dated at the university—a wonderfully warm, huggable blond—when she rushed a sorority. I took her decision to rush as a vow to live the unexamined life. I was stunned the next fall when I returned to campus to hear that she had died that summer bicycling in Germany. Going down a steep hill, she hadn't been able to stop and had crashed head first into a rock. I couldn't digest how this girl I had so glibly consigned to the lasting superficial bliss of the suburbs could die so young. It was I, the romantic poet, who was supposed to die young.

I fell in love with another girl at first sight when I was a freshman. She was too beautiful to ask out. Tall, with slender, Botticelli-like grace, she sat behind me in the main lecture hall of my contemporary philosophy class. I often looked back at her during lectures on Dewey, Ayer, Tillich, and Sartre philosophies (proving I hadn't lost my reason altogether). She wore off-beat dark wool clothes and had a dark bone comb perched as a crown in her tall generous fair hair. Her elegant bearing made her profoundly sensuous and regal.

During the following years at the university, I watched the Beatrice I never dared approach deteriorate. Her graceful slenderness was replaced by a haggard condition of being thin and run down. Her angelic white complexion turned pasty. She who had once defined her surroundings now appeared to be defined by whatever it was that surrounded her and brought her down. Drugs, alcohol, sleeping around—I didn't know what, but something had robbed her of her grace. One day when I was a graduating senior, I ran into her in front of a restaurant. I impulsively invited her to have coffee with me. She accepted. At the end of our faltering and clumsy conversation, she told me that her philosophy was that everyone should do what they wanted. She asked whether I agreed. I dissented mildly, while inside I violently disagreed. No one so beautiful should live by such an ugly idea. I wanted to scream out, No! See what this stupid idea has done to you. After fumbling my way to the end of our tattered conversation, I left the restaurant feeling sad. An angel had fallen, and my heart suffered a blow.

Sharply adding to my isolation was the fact that no sooner did I arrive at the university than I gave up going to church. I even played for a few months with the idea that I, a student who had barely passed freshman English, would write a book proving that Christianity was a false religion. In it I would argue that Christ was a creation of human needs. Unwittingly, I embraced one of atheism's oldest ideas as original with me.

I was truly a solitary rebel. I hung with no crowd and had no music, art, theater, drugs, clothing, or hairstyle by which to define myself. I found no substitute religion for the Catholicism I had rejected. I met one self-proclaimed Buddhist who looked as miserably lonely as the small dark room he inhabited.

The core of my painful solitude was my unceasing self-consciousness. Almost every day I faced the morning mirror resigned to the melancholy chore of having to think again this day, all day, about myself. My mind was a terrible prankster and a humiliator. It wouldn't allow me to be at ease with myself—not even for an hour. The more I sought to think myself free of myself, the more I thought about my thinking. I was a disturbed soul, a dog chasing its own tail. Consciousness was poisoning my heart, and there was no operation for this malady.

✎

The first relief I received from this infernal self-consciousness came one evening at the end of my sophomore year. I had been on a long study-date with a girl, one who was far more interested in studying than in sharing her affections with me. My frustration was fueled by my awareness that, over the past two months, I had forced myself to try to like her, even though in truth I was repulsed by her, especially her nervous habit of biting all her fingers until the tips were red and swollen. I left her at the door of her dormitory filled with intense frustration, loneliness, and self-disgust. On the way home, I knelt and prayed. I asked God to give me faith. After a while, I stood up believing in God.

I had undergone a conversion, a type of spiritual bypass. At the core, I had identified God with meaning, purpose, and love, all of which were stronger than my senses of isolation and futility. With this faith came hope that God would deliver me from myself. Prayer became an alternative to self-reflection. I accepted the agony of my mind as my cross. My terrible subjectivity had been pierced.

One Sunday, a month or so after my conversion, two Catholic scholars from the house invited me to go to mass with them. I experienced no special feeling at mass, but I emerged from the church ready to be a practicing Catholic. Of course, I knew a chasm stood between me and the church. I believed so little, and it taught so much. Yet my childhood familiarity with the church's doctrine and practice allowed me to accept it as my own.

Later that year I had another distinct religious experience. One evening, alone in the church, I prayed to Mary on behalf of all others. I shivered physically, experiencing what I took to be a veritable infusion of grace. I prayed without effort. The more I prayed the better I felt. As never before or since, I felt keenly that we humans are spiritually linked to one another beyond all divisions. Kneeling there in the church I experienced a change of heart.

Faith did not bring my mind and body to obedience, however. I still had to drag myself to mass. Once there, despite my best intentions, my mind wandered off in all sorts of directions. Even though I drenched myself with religious and spiritual reading, that did not quench all the sparks of my skepticism. Nor did faith still the desires of my flesh. I still hoped to meet someone I could love, marry and live with, body to body, heart to heart.

My conversion returned me to the faith of my family. I felt joined to what I took to be my mother's, father's, and grandparents' deepest hopes. I believed that I now truly belonged to the heart of the family. With prayer tying together the living and the dead, I could tend the family hearth.

The church also provided me—an uneducated neighborhood ethnic boy—with universality. It furnished a bridge between my family and all other Catholic peoples, especially peasants and workers. It offered a tradition not limited by time or place. It joined me to the vast and diverse history of Catholic thought. Behind me stood such great church fathers and doctors as Augustine, Aquinas, and Anselm. Finally, as Professor Tonsor would make clear to me, the church accorded me full access to Medieval Europe and European intellectual and cultural life.

∼※∽

I arrived at Stephen Tonsor's house, not having been there for a couple of years, to enact a familiar ritual. Even though I had visited his home infrequently, it felt like visiting a relative. Caroline, his wife, warmly welcomed me. She asked me about my wife, my children, and work. I replied with compliments on the beautiful plants that filled the living room and questions about her, her children, and her grandchildren. We discussed our aging mothers before she went off to the kitchen to finish preparing the large meal she invariably made for all my visits. Stephen, who had grown slightly heavier, sat in the same recliner flanked by stacks of book and articles on which he was at work.

After discussing shared acquaintances from my days at the university, we settled into a conversation about the condition of contemporary intellectual and academic life. All in all, my two hours with them were a delight. They both had plentiful enthusiasm. Age had not diminished his knowledge, or slackened his willingness to consider and judge the topic at hand. As I drove back to my motel afterward, I felt older and closer to death than my thriving mentor. At the same time, I felt privileged to have been again in the presence of my learned and kind mentor, even if this was to be the last time. He had returned me to my faith, advanced me in intellectual thought, and given me hope that my heart need not be forever divided.

I discovered history professor Stephen Tonsor as my first intellectual mentor in the fall semester of my junior year. An intellectually precocious friend, Renato Gonzalez, told me to take Tonsor's two-semester course on historiography, which amounted to a year-long history of history. Renato emphasized that Tonsor was a practicing Catholic.

In large part, Tonsor the man remained hidden behind his seriousness. His speaking style was restrained. He was rarely humorous. Banter was not one of his arts. In class, he never revealed anything about his personal life, with one exception. One day toward the end of the class period, out of the blue, he blurted out, as if making a confession, how painful it is to be hated by someone you love. Even in his office, Tonsor's manners were stiff. Yet he was most generous with his opinions and his books. He spoke in short declarative sentences that were always to the point. He responded to my fumbling questions with a straightforward instruction to acquaint myself with a certain book. I always left his office with a book or two under my arm. I immediately read them and promptly returned them in hopes of another conversation.

Like a couple that never learns to dance together, Tonsor and I carried on conversations that jerked and halted along. When I did dare assert something, he often replied by simply asserting the contrary. Once I argued that cataclysmic events define time. He retorted no, steady development does. I argued for volcanoes and earthquakes; he countered by describing the intellectual contribution of the nineteenth-century geologist Sir Charles Lyell, who demonstrated that long, slow geologic processes shaped the earth.

I took the few personal comments Tonsor made to me to heart. Once, addressing my proclivity for introspective questioning, he chided me. A plant can't grow if you continually pull it up and look at its roots, he said. Even though my introspection continued—it was a horse I had ridden too long to quickly dismount—he helped me understand its uselessness and prepared me to abandon even my churning mind to God's redemption.

I intently studied the comments he wrote on my papers. On a paper on Socrates (which I saved), he wrote, "I found your paper most interesting—and I share many of its basic ideas. While I think that notions of eternity are important, I do not believe we should be morbid about death, man's fate, about man's significance. Certainly Socrates was not and certainly Jesus was not. The more abundant life so frequently spoken of in the gospels was physical as well as spiritual. . . . Don't despise the body too much or you may end up thinking too little of the soul. Respect death for what it is; a minor event in a long life. Don't make too much fuss about it." I didn't understand the comment when he wrote it; I certainly didn't share his view as I approached my bypass.

Tonsor honored me when he called me into his office to discuss my paper on twentieth-century Spanish thinker Ortega y Gasset. In it I had argued that Ortega's hope of offering a new historicist liberal culture was vitiated at its heart by his failure to take into account the place of death in human experience. Tonsor wondered out loud if I had copied my paper, which he believed could not have been written by a student. He concluded, talking more to himself than to me, that the paper's poor English (especially my confused use of past participles) was proof enough that I did indeed write it.

What occurred inside his classroom changed my view of life. The first thing Tonsor did each day when he entered the room was to write on the board a bibliography of five to ten recommended books, a few of which were always in German. With no introductory pleasantries, Tonsor started to read his lecture. Each lecture focused on a thinker or a school of thinkers that ranged from Greek and Christian historians and philosophers to Enlightenment philosophers to romantics, positivists, and contemporary historians.

Under what I took to be the daunting German word *Weltanschauung* (which in English we translate as the diminished "world view"), Tonsor showed how historians express the views of an age. In both its most primitive and sophisticated forms, history reveals human attempts to attribute meaning to change. I understood the thrust of his argument to be that humanity, bound by time and caught amid events, is compelled to resort to myths and metaphors to make sense of its experience. It served my own apologetic interests to read Tonsor's implicit argument to be that scientific views depend as much on myth and metaphor as do religious views. (I recall Tonsor arguing that Gibbon's *Decline and Fall of the Roman Empire* depended as much on a consistent denial of miracles as Christian descriptions of this epoch depended on a belief in miracles.)

By my senior year, thanks to Tonsor and a range of important religious thinkers he recommended, I started to argue that primitive religions sought, above all else, wholeness and renewal. I identified this search with the core quest of my own inner life. I argued that through dance and myth, primitives sought the order, health, well-being, and fecundity that contemporary scientific and secular thought cannot satisfy.

This quest for salvation, I argued, worked itself out within the human heart beneath the surface of human history. I believed that as humanity went through time, its yearnings differentiated themselves around three different poles: the self, the other, and God. I conjectured that the advance of civilization increasingly transformed these poles into irreconcilable ends: The self culminated in the subjective and hedonistic individual; the other took its fullest form in conformist society and the all-powerful totalitarian nation-state; and God became a sheer idea divorced from nature, tribe, and even religious practice, a mere postulate of logical argumentation. Not one of the three—self, other, or God—met the individual's hunger for health and wholeness. Only the incarnate Christ could do that.

In the notes outlining my magnum opus, I drew an occasional graph of cones and triangles with self, other, and God at their poles. I concluded that only Jesus Christ—God and man, crucified redeemer—provided a redeeming truth, which must be a truth of heart. Christ alone offered a fecund, universal, and personal salvation myth for an age drawn and quartered by individualism, statism, and philosophical deisms. With primitive faiths shattered and with no order of personal and communal hope surviving, Christ alone—so I concluded—promised a true spring of springs, joining truth and the human hunger for salvation.

I continued to be obsessed with my grandiose philosophy of history even when I was out of the university and living at home and teaching high school history. In the spring of 1961, I even spread out all my notes on the basement Ping-Pong table to begin a sketch of my theology of history. More than once, I emerged from my work in the basement only to have my mother remind me that I still wasn't married and hadn't yet produced any grandchildren. University education had ruined me. Even though I had a legitimate job and had 175 high school students under my control, I still slept alone. It was clear—no matter what I claimed Tonsor did for me—that I spent more time with books than any normal young man should.

Embodiments

Homeward bound from my three days in Michigan, my thoughts turned from boyhood to the present. I flew to Minneapolis and then drove the remaining one hundred and fifty miles to Marshall, Minnesota, a small town in the western part of the state, mainly preoccupied with the operation that loomed ahead and the farewells I must bid my wife, my mother, and my four children.

Cathy, my wife, was my second heart. She had come to define my very senses. During twenty-seven years of marriage she had muted some emotions and let others flow for the first time. She had taken me from the iciness of mind and returned me to the warmth of flesh. She was the woman I sought, the body I needed.

Her movement and voice had come to mean home. She was the one around whom my arms fit best, the one who defined the life that embraced me. She was the one I had gotten used to. And now I felt I had to say—at least provisionally—farewell to her, the person I loved most.

In August 1966 we exited church doors in Rochester, New York, to Handel's "Water Music." Our recessional down that aisle concluded more than a year of walking—walking and hugging, walking and talking, walking and deciding. We walked around the university, where Cathy was completing a B.S. in nursing and I a Ph.D. in history. We walked deep into the large urban park through which the Genesee River ran and whose opening faced the university, comforting each other about our studies, her trying work shifts, and even our mutual fears of nuclear war. We walked on the large asylum grounds that bordered her apartment. We walked up into brush lands behind my apartment in the hills of Binghamton, New York, where I taught for a semester before taking my doctoral examinations. And we walked the trails around Toughannock Falls and down along the banks of Lake Cayuga, where I booked myself into a cabin for two weeks to prepare for my examinations in Enlightenment history.

Cathy and I seemed meant for each other. The small things we did together became memorable, as they do for those in love. Once she got her old ice skates out—the leather on them was cracked and they were losing their color—and with stiff legs, hesitantly, she let me guide her around a frozen pond. When she tired, I glided over the pond in great circles, showing off.

Cathy did not value words and talking as I did, and that was good. In fact, it was crucial. She didn't tease or taunt, which I wouldn't have liked—I always took things so much to heart. She didn't hide herself in enigmatic or sullen moods or ask me to come looking for her. And she never once during our courtship pressed me to say what was on my mind. If she had, doubtless we would have thrown our relationship into the maelstrom of my subjectivity. From painful experience I knew that certain things can't and shouldn't be said because, as momentary and fleeting as they are, they won't and can't be forgotten; and other things can't be talked about because they aren't certain. Cathy never confused words with real things, or changing feelings with the depths of the human heart.

Cathy worked as a public health nurse in downtown Philadelphia before coming to Rochester, New York. Nurses were in my family, and I believed they made good wives. I probably gained my reasoning from my mother, and it ran thus: If a woman is altruistic enough to nurse strangers, she will lavish even more care on her own family. I was also attracted to nurses because I felt they knew what I didn't: They saw people being born and dying, and they tried to heal them.

As so often happens with couples, coincidence played a role in getting and keeping us together. We met in the hospital cafeteria, where I happened to eat one day. After supper, we took a walk. Finding out that she was from Pennsylvania, I described the Pennsylvania village I had visited as a boy. I didn't recall its name (Kelayres), but I remembered its dirt-covered streets on which my cousins played bocce ball. Cathy told me her hometown, McAdoo, was right next door. I then distinctly remembered walking the road from Kelayres to McAdoo one evening on the way to McAdoo's town fair. She knew my relatives. Her father's parents had immigrated from Galicia and arrived at the same place my father's parents landed when they immigrated from Sicily.

Before I fell in love with Cathy, I had studied Spanish and traveled in Mexico, believing I shared a special affinity with Spanish culture. Then I learned Russian, more or less believing I had a special identity with the Russian people's literature and soul. Next I learned French and studied for my master's in history in Quebec, at the Université de Laval, believing that I had an affinity with French culture. Each time I expected to find home and didn't. Here, in Cathy's land, the anthracite coal region, where Italians and Slavs struggled to make themselves at home, I found my people.

Another coincidence proved to be important. At one point we had broken off our relationship, no longer believing things could be worked out, mostly because of my dark moods. After a short trip to Binghamton, I returned to Rochester and attended mass, hoping to see Cathy. She was there, and I took this to be a sign that we were meant for one another.

Still, I fretted at the prospect of marriage far more than I worried now about my pending bypass. Marriage, I knew, meant a whole lifetime. And a lifetime, whatever that was, struck me as a serious matter. I projected my worst fears into the future. I feared that marriage would freeze me in ice. Into my dreams of Cathy and me in a bodily community crept images of myself as Dostoevsky's Underground Man. My mind taunted me. Even after buying her a ring and ordering a cake, I moved the date of our wedding back two months to mollify my doubts. I had to battle my way to the altar far more fiercely than I did into elective heart surgery.

We sought counseling from a local priest named Father Kurtz. He told me my reservations were natural. Attempting to comfort me, he suggested that I had only one problem: "getting along with other people." After our last counseling session, he took Cathy and me for a flight in his airplane. Near the end of our flight, he drove the plane straight up into a stall and then dropped. Unwarned in advance of this stunt, Cathy was terrified. And I was delighted in falling through the sky. We did not treat it as sign of things to come, but an experience not to be forgotten.

We walked out of his church married and happy. We spent our first days and nights together crossing the country in our 1965 Volkswagen and sleeping in the new tent we had bought. After a small celebration of family and friends in the yard of the house where Cathy lived with four other nurses, we left Rochester for Cathy's home in northeast Pennsylvania. From there we drove to Detroit, visiting some of her relatives along the way. My parents threw us a large wedding party in their backyard, where we camped out for our four-day stay, amusing relatives and neighbors.

Early on the fifth morning we piled everything we owned, which was very little, into our little green Volkswagen, setting out for Riverside, California, where I had an instructorship teaching Western civilization. Too romantic to drive expressways all the way to California, we took to state and county roads just past Chicago. After visiting the House on the Rock in Wisconsin, we crossed the Mississippi River at La Crosse. At one point in the interminable cornfields of southern Minnesota—not far from where we have lived for more than twenty-five years now—I distinctly remember declaring to Cathy, "God, how awful it would be to be stuck out in one of these little towns surrounded by endless fields of corn."

At Grand Teton National Park, we enrolled, as a lark, in mountain-climbing school, convinced that the school was more about entertaining tourists than about true mountain climbing. However, after a short boat trip and instructions on how to tie a bowline knot, things quickly turned serious. On slippery surfaces, we sought nonexistent toeholds and footholds. From a sole piton, we swung out off the sides of a mountain above valleys below. The last move of the day, which required us to rappel off a hundred-foot cliff, was a near disaster for Cathy. On her descent, she got out of rhythm. Rather than make a small release of the rope and a gentle bounce with her feet over the cliff's side, she descended by jerks, releasing either too little or too much rope: Twisting and twirling, jerking and bumping, she descended the cliff. She landed on the ground unhurt, but crying. I was filled with guilt. I had almost killed my bride. We didn't wait around to see if we passed the first day of mountain-climbing school.

We entered southern California and traveled through the desert on our way to Riverside, a desert town that we instantly liked. Though arid and defined by constant blue skies under which grasses and vegetation were always on the verge of turning brown, Riverside was a feast of vivid colors. Everything seemed to grow there. Surrounded by orange groves, the city boasted streets lined with palms and homes adorned with multiple bushes and flowers. Its quaint downtown was built around the fantasy-like Mission Inn. From our rented house at the edge of Riverside's city park, which was centered around a large artificial lake, we had views of the distant Mt. San Gorgonio and Mt. San Jacinto—when weather and smog permitted.

Cathy made a home for us in Riverside out of our simple and meager belongings. She shopped, cooked wonderful meals (which undoubtedly contributed to the fifteen pounds I gained during our first year of marriage), wrote letters, picked bouquets of flowers, and sewed bright red floral curtains. She filled the space around her with pleasantness. Her voice was full, smooth, and reassuring. She moved with a graceful gait that I found neither too fast nor too slow. Blessed with good health, she made herself attractive without being vainly self-preoccupied. She was pleased by small things—a hike into the nearby hills, a Sunday trip to the ocean—and she was willing to go along with most anything, at least when asked a second time.

Soon, only a few months after our marriage, she was pregnant with one of the eight or ten children we planned to have. Our days were measured by her swelling stomach, the movement of life within her, and the appearance of our first-born, Felice. In the middle of the night we rushed to the hospital, where I stood vigil again for another turning point in our lives. Then, twenty hours later, after a long labor, Felice was born; big and red, with her hair standing straight up, she appeared terrifyingly awake. And awake is how Cathy and I spent our first year of parenthood. Neither Cathy's milk nor our rocking could quiet Felice during the long nights of that first year.

Our lives revolved around Felice, but we still managed time for entertaining new acquaintances and friends. We also traveled and explored the region, driving up into the mountains, down to the ocean, and out into the desert. A few times we visited my grandmother Rosalia's godmother, or *cummari*, Rosalia Brucato, in nearby Ontario, California. (The term *cummari* in this case described the close friendship she and my grandmother had in the old days in Detroit when my grandmother was alone with her children.) After the Second World War, Rosalia and her family left Detroit for California, their new Sicily, where they set up a successful chicken farm. Rosalia lived alone in a large ranch home at the front of her property with her daughter, Lina, and her husband Fred, who suffered from advanced emphysema brought on by years of working with dusty chickens.

At Rosalia Brucato's home, as at my grandmother's, what mattered was talk, hands at work, and food. Bountiful produce from the garden kept Lina and Rosalia busy under their plastic-covered back porch and around their kitchen table, the two places where they spent most of their waking hours. The living room and dining room, whose furniture was covered by plastic drop clothes, were reserved for baptisms, deaths, and other very special occasions. Rosalia, small, heavy, and highly animated, with light skin and dark flashing eyes, reminded me so much of my grandmother. But I never visited Rosalia and her family without sensing my grandmother's jealousy in the afterlife: She was dead, and here was her *cummari,* Rosalia, alive and holding her only son's only son's first child.

⌗

Marriage treated me well. It was a connecting sacrament. It provided someone to come home to. It made our repetitious days comfortably familiar. A good woman makes a good marriage, and a good marriage makes a good home.

Yet marriage did not completely disarm the icy demons within me. I still had days when I felt alone, a prisoner of distancing consciousness. I often prayed to God that I would be free of them.

Help came in the person of "Morty," a philosophy instructor at the university. He was at work on a doctoral dissertation that would combine existential phenomenology with traditional Indian attempts to transcend the self. But that is not what attracted me. Rather, Morty, as no one else I had ever heard before, directly confronted the radical wantonness of our thoughts and feelings. His favorite analogy was that our minds are like a living room. People enter it, sit down, and say all sorts of things: things that get our goat, anger us, belittle our character, and awaken our fears. When they say things we don't like, we argue with them. The more we argue, the longer they stay and the louder and more obnoxious they become. And, if, out of frustration, we try to throw them out altogether, they become stronger yet. We can do nothing to free ourselves from their unwanted conversations, unless—and this was the hopeful part of Morty's message that attracted me—we listen quietly and fully to them. We must let them have their full say about everything, and never once interrupt or argue with them. Once we have truly heard these voices out, the unwanted visitors of our mind, Morty promised, will leave of their own accord. And, in time, as we learn to listen to them, their stays will be shorter and less unpleasant, until they have lost all power over us.

Morty's promise held. His freeing insights remained with me. Even as I prepared for open heart surgery, I knew that though the risk of death was real, the fears bypass awoke were illusions. I welcomed these strangers into my consciousness without resistance, only to send them packing as soon as I knew that their powers to control were only as potent as the reality I attributed to them.

Morty and I visited one another. His small, minimally furnished apartment squared with his life as bachelor and thinker, but it struck me with a sense of paucity. At one of the sessions that he held in his apartment, a couple of months after I had met him, we locked horns. When he was through with his talk, I asked him, What is the difference between the consciousness that hears and reacts and the consciousness that listens and goes beyond? First he ignored my question. Then he gave an insufficient answer, and when I persisted, he became angry and insulting. I left his apartment confident that he was still in the valley of the self and alone, and that I was far better off with a wife, a child, and red floral curtains.

The Vietnam War also reconnected me to the world. It was another kind of bypass out of self back to community, action, politics, and commitment. Before the war I was consistently and, to a degree, arrogantly apolitical. However, as an instructor at the University of New York in Binghamton in 1965 and 1966, I was daily given a copy of the *New York Times*—and what little I read there, and in *Ramparts,* persuaded me that the nation was miring itself in a losing jungle war. The more supporters of the war defended it, the more apparent it became to me that this was our Syracusan Expedition — the time when our blood boiled hot, when presumption and honor sacrificed fresh young lives and old and better ways.

Already by the time we reached California, in late summer of 1966, I judged the war to be insanity. Cathy and I started to protest it. First, another professor and I led a group of sixty people out to March Air Force Base, where we practiced dying while they simulated a nuclear attack. Then I organized a death march of one hundred individuals (including children) to protest at March Air Force Base when it celebrated its fiftieth anniversary. We also protested at the downtown mall and in front of the draft board offices. We have a photograph showing Cathy, pregnant with Tony, our first son, carrying a sign that indicated that she practiced what she preached: Make love, not war. We conducted a five-day hunger strike at the university and took a trip to the Los Angeles federal courthouse, where I joined a few hundred others in openly supporting those who resisted the draft. I also wrote to my own draft board, telling them that as long as the nation had nuclear weapons and was fighting the war in Vietnam, they should understand that I would not serve.

Protest was exhilarating and self-dramatizing. Believing intensely that I was right and acting accordingly caused me to take a great leap from political indifference to public risk. I, who just a few years before had been locked within the turnings of my own mind, protested openly in the streets and was written about in the newspaper. I was a protester and proud of it. Our photographs were taken repeatedly by the military security. At one point we believed our telephone was tapped. We were attacked in letters to the editor.

Bearing witness against the war took me out of the security of the home I had just found. It threatened my career and activated my conscience. It led me onto a fresh moral ground where courage counted most and self was transformed by commitment and action. It was as if I had been given a new heart, suffused with oxygen-rich blood, that believed in bearing public witness to the world.

Opposition to the war turned us outward. With marginal faith and minimal efforts, Cathy and I supported the founding of a local chapter of the Peace and Freedom Party. We did our best to see that two of my African-American students were elected officers. We went north to show our support for Cesar Chavez and the Delano Valley grape workers. We helped register voters in Riverside for Robert Kennedy even though I leaned toward Gene McCarthy, the candidate who refused to be a candidate. The world of 1968 (starting with the Tet Offensive, followed by Johnson's decision not to seek the presidency, and dramatized by Martin Luther King's assassination) exploded with horror, surprises, and possibilities. We felt as if we verged on a historical turning point.

Protest brought us new friends. We associated with activist Christians and especially Catholics, several of whom were identified with the Catholic Worker Movement, which since the 1930s had identified with the poor and the political left and embraced pacifism during the Second World War. We were fond of Jack and Mary Thorton, whom we idealized. Almost two decades older than us, silver-haired Jack and good-hearted Mary appeared to be living the committed Christian life we intended to live. They had met while serving on a soup line at the Catholic Worker in the Bowery. They were personal friends with Dorothy Day, Peter Maurin, and Ammon Hennesey, who protested, boycotted, and picketed as much as any person in American history. While I didn't share their thorough-going conscientious objector views, I respected the way he and Mary lived their beliefs. They had started a small farm in Pennsylvania whose doors they opened to neighbors and recently released prisoners until bad times led their family of ten or so, which later would expand to fifteen, to California, where Jack earned a living as a secondary teacher. There he discovered, as we all do, that people don't live by ideas and good intentions alone.

With their example before us, Cathy and I took up the Catholic Worker ideal. We would produce a large and loving family and, at the same time, pay the price of communal and political involvement: We would act out of conscience, even if it meant jail or exile. In contrast to Morty's teaching, we would seek not the good in psychological liberation but imitation of the incarnate Christ.

Analyzing this ideal was a primary object of my dissertation. In making a critical historical examination of Emmanuel Mounier's personalism, I would examine many of the principles and experiences that defined the Catholic Worker ideal. From the late 1920s until his premature death in 1950, Mounier stressed that the human person is a spiritual creature who is embodied in and responsible for community. Mounier articulated his personalism in reference to opposing poles. In contrast to the narrow, selfish, material individual, the person completes himself by engagement in community. In opposition to abstract, mass, economic, and totalitarian society, the personalist community seeks to fulfill individual and group, matter and spirit, action and values.

By the end of May 1968, I was ready to return east to begin my doctoral studies. I needed a period of meditative regathering—a *recueillement,* to use Mounier's own phrase. Protest wore me out—the strain of worrying when the Selective Service System might come knocking at our door, the sharp recognition that our local nonviolent protest would not make a difference. Expanding or stopping the war turned on large events and the outcome of national politics, especially the election of a new president. Bobby Kennedy's assassination did not bode well.

I was ready for the sidelines, and so was Cathy. She was pregnant again, and it was time to get the dissertation out of the way and find a job.

Incarnations

I continued thinking about the first years of marriage, when heart and body came together again after having been disassociated in adolescence. As the day of surgery drew pressingly near, I pulled more of my past into my present. I set it in front of me to leave it behind me. The days became a time of judgments and farewells, as if I were lightening myself for a great crossing.

Life had packed my heart; now, I was unpacking it, possibly for the last time. I unpacked gently, surrendering myself to God's mercy, knowing that finally it fell to him to sort out what my heart had recorded.

⚬—⚭

We left California, where the beaches were occupied with fair immortal youth, for the more mortal and corpulent beaches of the East Coast, where people had cancer and heart problems. There we were more at home. Cathy was eight months pregnant with our second child, Tony. And thanks to her good cooking and my inactivity, I was twenty-five pounds heavier. Still smoking, I was no doubt well along the road to heart disease.

We tried to live at the Catholic Worker community on the banks of the Hudson River at Tivoli, New York, but it was not a good place for a young family. Then my plans for Cathy and the children to join me in France, where I was at my work on my dissertation, failed. I returned from France after two months, and we spent the rest of a long, difficult year alternating between living with my folks in East Detroit and hers in McAdoo.

While at Cathy's parents' home, I escaped the hubbub of family life every day to work in the back room of her father's law office. The two-story brick and tin-sided Bavolack Building testified to her paternal grandparents' success as grocers. They had escaped the mines, which her mother's parents had not. Cathy's father, Adam, made me at home in the small room. I browsed in the law digests and reference books set in glass-windowed oak book cases. I liked the feel of old things in the office—the textbooks from the twenties, the high tin ceiling, the Tiffany lamp.

Adam introduced me to the village of which he was burgess for twenty years and the region in which he had done politics for even longer. He picked up on my interest in law. When job possibilities appeared exhausted in the spring of 1969, he generously offered to pay my way through law school. Adam served as the top Schuylkill County assistant district attorney, and a few of his legal briefs had reached the Pennsylvania Supreme Court.

Adam was also fifty to sixty pounds overweight. Hardly the picture of good health, he indulged himself with evening snacking and smoking. He battled frequent colds and flu with over-the-counter medicines. Yet his infirmities were superficial. Though generous, Adam could be tough and nagging, determined and proud. He had remarkable energy for a man in his late sixties. He led the church choir, played pool, went to the YMCA in Hazelton, and played golf. He was always on the go. Even at the end of the day, which didn't occur until 10:00 P.M. after evening sessions at his office, he would return home to prepare a case or annoyingly read aloud to whoever was around whatever he found interesting in the newspaper.

I mistakenly measured my health against Adam's. I assured myself that I would be in better condition than he was when I was his age. If a man so overweight and still smoking could live so long and so well, so could I. But I didn't entirely believe myself. There was a determination about Adam that made me sense my mortality when I was around him. He seemed more embedded in life than I was. More ethereal, I felt vulnerable to my subjectivity.

Adam was embedded in his place. As a county attorney, member of the Lions Club, active Republican, and burgess, he fully participated in community life. He subordinated his family to the interests of locale, which embittered his wife. She had come from a mining family of twelve children far poorer than Adam's. Nevertheless, her family had succeeded every bit as much as Adam's. Yet, she contended, his family got the glory and praise and, worse, acted as if it were superior, especially when Adam's relatives flaunted their Ukrainian identity.

Once in a while, Catherine would tell me that Adam never bought her a nice house of which she could be proud. As a child she had hidden in slag heaps so that other children wouldn't see how poorly she was dressed. She begged for leftover food from miners coming up from the mines at the end of the day. She helped support the family, went to school, became a teacher, and continued to support her family until she married in her thirties.

When her two girls were raised, Catherine returned to work as a teacher. Still Adam didn't buy her a new home. They lived in an outdated two-story duplex, which no amount of fixing up could turn into the nice house Catherine wanted. Adam would not budge on this issue. He could never see the benefit of a new house, while each year Catherine saw her friends, whose husbands weren't professionals, move into spacious new homes.

For the most part, Catherine's resentment bounced off Adam. It didn't deflect him from his daily rounds, on which he often took me. He introduced me to his clients and lawyer friends at the Pottsville Country Club. He showed me around the courthouse, where in his sixties he finally began to serve as the first county attorney, having long since paid his dues to the Republican "English machine."

As protest in California taught me one kind of politics, Adam taught me another: the local politics of Pennsylvania. It was an ongoing, mundane politics of ethnic groups and friends; it turned on gifts, reciprocities, and jobs on the turnpike and in Harrisburg. Adam explained why the widow got her coal bin filled in the fall and why the drunk got his drink on election day. Adam clearly understood how his own ethnic group, the Carpatho-Rusyns (a small group of rural folk from the Carpathian Mountains), were defined only after their arrival in the United States. He understood how churches (Orthodox and Catholic) and nationalists (especially Ukrainians) warred in this country over the identities and loyalties of these transplanted mountain peasants. Thanks to Adam, I—who knew myself to be my own invention—discovered that groups, which can take things personally and to heart, are also artificial and recent inventions.

Adam outlined for me the political path that finally led him to his position as county district attorney. When Adam started law, he knew he had to choose a party to succeed; he became a Republican. He knew that the Irish—who were the Democrats—weren't giving anything (other than beatings) to the Slavs or Italians. So, like my Sicilian cousins in nearby Kelayres, Adam accepted the scraps that fell from the English/Welsh Republican table. From his freshman days at Bucknell, he knew "the English" weren't friends of Catholics and Slavs, but he also knew that they needed to beat the rival Irish Democratic machine. Away from the political arena, Adam was most comfortable with fellow Slavs and Italians.

As the country was swept up in the conflagration of national events, Adam explained to me the local fires. I learned about the Irish Molly McGuires who organized the early Irish miners. Their trials were held in the very courthouse where Adam practiced law. I learned that the fated Lattimore strikers started their march in McAdoo, on the street where Adam and Catherine lived. Adam gave me a book on neighboring Kelayres, the adjacent village where my grandparents from Sicily first lived, which described how in 1934 members of the Bruno clan (officially identified with the Republican party) killed five Democrats and wounded another twenty who were parading in support of a candidate intent on removing the Brunos from office.

The more I knew of the region, the more I took it to heart. I liked its politics and its diverse and coarse-voiced working-class peoples. They weren't educated or rich enough to disguise their peasant backgrounds—and I liked them for it. One old man in Kelayres, Tony DiMaria, told me stories about events that occurred when my grandfather was young.

I felt at home on this broken landscape. It resonated with the mortality I associated with life, and thus spoke to my heart. The small towns were set atop mountains or nestled in valleys. Small, well-kept patches of life, they seemed menaced by open mining pits and slag heaps that only reluctantly yielded vegetation. There was plenty in the anthracite region of Pennsylvania for ecologists to despise. Here the skin had been torn off the earth. The pockmarked landscape offered a ready-made landfill for anyone who had anything to dump. Even Philadelphia proposed filling old mines with its garbage. Nobody thought about the region's groundwater. A crack in someone's basement in Coal Dale opened a two-hundred-foot crevice to the mines below. In several places in the region, underground fires in coal veins burned for decades, causing occasional evacuations of towns. Coal dust remained everywhere, testifying to both the birth and death of king coal.

The coal region reinforced my view of life. People get old and die. Nobody can, or finally cares to, keep up with the most recent fashions in appearance or thought. Nothing humans do is pure. Progress always has a price, and community exists only in patches. Yet as much as I took to this region and enjoyed kicking about with Adam, I didn't accept his offer to pay my way through law school. Accepting it would have meant another three or four years of study and a lifetime of indebtedness. Besides, I had invested too much in history to so quickly abandon it.

I was particularly committed to my dissertation topic, which I wrote under the kindness and intelligence of my second mentor, A. W. Salomone of the University of Rochester. It furnished a way for me to seek a relevant Christian philosophy for our times. I took pride in my new-found critical prowess, which rested on the notion that man—at least intellectual man—does live by words alone; metaphors and myths matter to him more than experiences do. My central argument was that Mounier was an intellectual, as I ambivalently took myself to be. Despite his personalist manifesto's commitment to be embodied and act in this century, his philosophy was ruled by the principles of nineteenth-century Catholic social thought. Even though his personalism affirmed that Western civilization had entered a profound crisis and that embodied man must live and react amidst circumstances, Mounier and his generation did not understand power and diplomacy. They totally failed to grasp the events leading to the Second World War. He and those gathered around personalism and the journal *Esprit* only began to recognize the true dimensions of things when Poland fell and German tanks crossed French borders. Even after the war, he persisted in his debilitating love of intellectual symmetry. It caused him to treat communist Russia and capitalist United States as twin evils, as French intellectuals fashionably did. I concluded that his personalism, in the end, constituted an elaborate attempt to remain loyal to nineteenth-century Catholic communitarianism in a cruelly noncommunal century. Mounier himself was another intellectual who preferred theory to fact.

The gulf between ideals and power was confirmed for me by the events of 1968. The events of that year convinced me that I would not accomplish much as a protester on the streets or in political caucuses, and that I would be better off staying home with my family and writing my dissertation. The debacle of the Democratic Convention in Chicago was the emphatic and culminating lesson. I stayed up late on my parents' back porch watching the police riot against the crowds. This outcome had been predictable from the moment the protesters assembled leaderless in Chicago. They went there with no plan or leadership. They were in Chicago "to make something happen." They did—and I was as pained by their moral failure as by the cruel blows of the police that fell upon them. I realized then that the war would not be stopped by protest.

Violence had outrun hope. 1968 was a year in which good hearts were defeated by silly ideas, unexpected events, and raw power, a year in which so many possibilities were envisioned and almost all the bad ones were realized.

The year wore a similar mask in Europe. The spring uprising of the French students, *les événements de mai,* had the delayed consequence of forcing the French President, Charles de Gaulle, to step down. In August, the well-known face of raw power was exposed as Soviet tanks crushed Czechoslovakian citizens. Prague's spring was over—and I, who had just discovered my need to be engaged in politics, was painfully instructed in the limits of action. Doing research in France in the fall of 1968, I heard at the Mounier community a group of Czech Protestant ministers tell a French personalist audience that their nation had undergone a real revolution in 1948. What had occurred in 1968 was a mere setback. I told them they had their 48s wrong. They had failed to gain independence in the revolution of 1848, and 1948 left them still bound by tyranny. They were still one revolution short of freedom. A week later in Paris, I listened to liberal Democrat Pierre Salinger (former friend and press secretary of President John F. Kennedy) explain to a French and American students why American draft protesters shouldn't receive amnesty even if they were right about the war being wrong. Still in Paris at the time of Nixon's election, I found myself repeating a worn French cliché: "The more it changes, the more it remains the same." No political bypass was offered, reminding me if only by analogy how tragedy goes with the course of things and serious heart surgery can mortally fail.

I returned home from France ready to write my dissertation and find a teaching job. I was surprised by a telephone call that came while I was working in my back room at Adam's office.

Maynard Brass, the head of the history program at a new college in southwestern Minnesota, asked if I would come out for an interview. Feeling abused and humiliated by how my job search had progressed that year, I agreed to come only on the condition that I not be asked to fly halfway across the nation only to be one of a parade of candidates. Maynard replied that the university wasn't interested in paying travel expenses for a candidate who wasn't interested in the job. I went for the interview.

─✽─

The brand new college's mission was as undefined as its campus, which amounted to a few buildings in a cornfield on the eastern end of a small rural town of five thousand in the heart of America. Almost every question I asked Maynard on the car ride from the Brooking's airport to Marshall drew the same response: "That will be for you to define." This was true even of a required freshman course entitled "Flux," which rhymed in my mind with a very popular word of the hour.

But many good things impressed me. I liked Maynard instantly. I was pleased with the nearby river valley state park he showed me on the way to the college. The chance for a tenured job was reasonably strong. At least, I could stay long enough to complete my dissertation and let Cathy and me catch up with ourselves before we returned to the east. I accepted the job. Cathy then, as before the bypass, was docile, accepting risk with as much equanimity as she accepted the repetition and travail of everyday life.

A few months later, in early August, we set out for Minnesota. We found ourselves again crossing the Mississippi, which in the intervening three years seemed to have grown much smaller. I am sure the Santa Barbara oil spill and the incident with nerve gas at Dugway proving ground had had an effect on me. A dawning ecological consciousness had irreversibly diminished the permanence and grandeur of nature. Awe of the mighty had been turned into concern for the fragile.

We bought a large old four-bedroom house on the east end of Main Street in the small village of Cottonwood, Minnesota. In that house (known originally as the Dahl House and then called the Catlin House, after the town's first banker) in that essentially Norwegian village of eight hundred, thirteen miles from Marshall, we began to weave our lives.

We had two more children, Adam and Ethel. We had a new roof put on the house, put in a new furnace, and peeled away seven layers of wallpaper that went back to the turn of the century. We walked the children along the village streets to the post office and to one of the dozen or so small stores that lined the two sides of Main Street. During the summer, we drove out to farms to see the animals (the children were thrilled by the hissing and attacking geese) and stayed at the town beach until the sun sank below the horizon. In the winter, we took the children skating on the lake or sledding on the short, steep banks of the nearby drainage ditch.

We shopped at local stores, including the Coast-to-Coast, where we were frequently told that the goods we wanted were "coming in on Thursday." We teased behind the proprietor's back that no doubt Christ's second coming was coming on Thursday's truck. We saw old Doctor Borgeson in nearby

Hanley Falls for our physicals and ailments. Borgeson resented the merciless insurance forms that accumulated in one giant mound on his dining room table. Aging rapidly, Borgeson missed the birth of our last child, Ethel, altogether. Cathy delivered Ethel with the help of a nurse and me. Borgeson arrived in time to carry out a lengthy and intricate episiotomy that left me sitting on the floor woozy.

Bess, the widow who lived next door, became the best of friends with our daughter Felice. Every evening for several years they watched *Little House on the Prairie*. Once a week they ate together. Mrs. Kleppie prepared their meal and came to think of us as such close neighbors that she entered our house without knocking.

Our children were never made to feel like outsiders. They fit in at school and played freely and safely wherever their adventures in town led them. They usually made home base an empty, weed-covered lot which they called "The Foundation." Felice, the self-appointed director of play, frequently organized her brothers and the neighborhood children into plays and group activities.

When he was four, our oldest son, Tony, decided he wanted to be a farmer and drive the impressive machinery that regularly rolled down our street. He wore cowboy boots and hat, and paid frequent visits to the local farm machinery lots, where he would climb up on tractors and combines. Later he and his brother, Adam, and their friends—and occasionally our youngest daughter, Ethel—played at the abandoned mink farm across the street, making its empty office their secret headquarters.

With her hands filled with young children, first two, then three, and finally four, and an old house to renovate, Cathy didn't need a village bigger than Cottonwood. Her days were full and comfortably routine. They amounted to a walk around town, a trip to the library, a visit with Bess or one of the other neighbors, or a weekly trip to Marshall to shop. Raised in a small town of a few thousand herself, she brought no great expectations to the everyday life of this ordinary village and, hence, suffered no disappointment or disillusionment.

While the bulk of my energy was focused at the university, I did not escape the predictable controversy that surrounds a college professor in a small town. In an atmosphere charged by debate over the Vietnam War, and by mounting student protests, it was nearly inevitable that I would be labeled an agitator and anti-American, especially after writing a letter to the editor of the *Marshall Independent* warning the region's youth not to trust their futures to the old "patriots" of the local draft boards. I became even more involved in controversy when a few other professors and I challenged the appropriateness of the local legion's placement of a World War II cannon in the town's new war memorial. The battle of the cannon resonated in the paper for weeks and in the coffee shops and bars long after the first shot had been fired. The conflict pitted the legionnaires' right to express their loyalty and gratitude to the fellow military dead against the professors' right to defend future generations against what they took to be the symbolic perpetration of war and death.

For seven years we made ourselves at home in a small town

on the prairie. We liked best the way people were connected to one another. Everybody who met in that small town knew somebody in common. We grew used to the prairie's shady villages and its grove-protected farms, and came to cherish the vast open spaces that surrounded them. We actually began to feel claustrophobic among mountains and in the woods. I even developed a grudging respect for the prairie's constant winds, which made golf a formidable test and ice-skating, at times, altogether impossible.

I openly revered the winters as if they were a badge of honor to be proudly worn. I enjoyed telling others of terrible blizzards that drove animals into the fields, iced over their nostrils, froze their breath, and then buried them in great mounds of snow. The wind and cold could turn the white fields into seas of frozen waves. The prairie connected death and ice, as did thoughts of my forthcoming bypass, which would stop my heart and, as if my chest were a cooler, pack it with ice. The very act of freezing to death and being buried in snow seemed, if one had to die—and one of my students did die that way— a sweet and gentle way to lose the warmth of life.

We went outdoors during the winter months whenever we could. We considered winter the first natural sacrament of our region and gleefully accepted the bragging rights it gave us when asked by outsiders how cold it gets "out there." Even on the coldest days, Cathy insisted that the children play outdoors at least for a while. Once, after a sudden blizzard, the children gathered and brought into the house sparrows frozen stiff. They put them in their Fisher-Price barn. When the birds revived, they flew all over the house. They were hope in the coldest of winters.

⚶

Down the road, at the new college, my days were full. Maynard and a colleague and I had to develop a history curriculum and help shape a social science requirement. I had brand-new courses to teach. I helped hire new colleagues, among whom numbered my lifelong friend Ted Radzilowski; David Nass, originally from Massachusetts, who became a dear friend; and Michael Kopp, who became a buddy during his stints at the college.

In addition to defining the university's curriculum, I became one of the architects of the institution. With a colleague I founded the Faculty Forum, the first institution of public debate on the campus. Considerable suspicion and acrimony surrounded it until it was institutionalized as the Faculty Senate.

Taking advantage of the 1971 Public Employees Labor Relations Act (PELRA), I formed a controversial local union whose goal was to form local (rather than statewide) bargaining units along with a statewide bargaining unit that excluded department chairs and administration. In our second year, the local union became affiliated with the Minnesota Federation of Teachers (MFT). Over the next several years we waged war on a number of battlefields. Statewide, our battle was against the company union, the Inter-Faculty Organization (IFO) and its supporter, the Minnesota Educational Association (MEA). The IFO had the numbers and the vision for a statewide unit, but it lacked intelligence and will. At home, we battled a precipitous decline in enrollment that took us from thirty-five hundred students in 1970 to about half that number by 1976, with corresponding losses of faculty that left us with only a hundred colleagues.

I loved the battle. I loved the strategy meetings, the trips across the state, and the never-ending telephone calls. I felt terribly alive. At stake was the fate of our college, our jobs, and the union. Unlike the Vietnam War protests, here I could actually influence outcomes, and I wasn't worried about winding up in jail. I smoked cigars. I got heavier from an evening diet of pizza and beer, the nourishment of choice at our union planning sessions. And there was no time for exercise. I felt important—and no doubt my heart was being injured by my passion for the union cause.

The speakers we brought to campus—Dorothy Day and Danilo Dolci among them—fit my notion of social justice. And they, in turn, provided encouragement to participate in other union causes. We picketed the local liquor store in support of the Cesar Chavez battle against California grape growers. We threatened to picket the local clothing store over a national dispute between garment makers and owners. Later we helped the striking bank women of Willmar, Minnesota, by writing small articles for *The Progressive*, fund-raising with the UAW-CIO, and picket-line walking. And, of course, we held war protests. When Nixon mined the ports of North Vietnam and invaded Cambodia, we nonviolently blocked the streets of Marshall. One hundred and sixty of us—a larger group than anywhere else in the nation—were arrested and spent the afternoon in jail. Like the farmers who shut down Marshall in the 1930s, we brought national issues to the heartland.

By the time I was given a sabbatical for the 1975–1976 academic year, I was exhausted. There had been little peace for me on this quiet corner of the prairie. Our union had been defeated; after several appeals, the Minnesota Supreme Court ordered a statewide unit. If I was worn out at school, Cathy was even more burdened at home. She breast-fed our four children until they were two or three. She formed the regional La Leche League. And somehow she found time to redecorate the house, attend political conventions, and nurse older neighbors. Our summer and Christmas vacations were not vacations for her or me. They were three-thousand-mile ordeals to Michigan, then Pennsylvania, then back to Michigan and home. At both our parents' houses, Cathy had to try to keep the children from upsetting the grandparents, particularly at my parents' home, where my father loved his rituals and my mother's mood swings were severe.

After Ethel's birth in 1973, Cathy openly admitted that she was exhausted. She had all the children she felt she could handle. We tried the church's prescriptions for birth control, but to no good effect. The pope, I took to saying, had never tried baby-sitting. Abstinence was out of the question. Cathy was afraid of the pill, and I concluded that a vasectomy was an easier operation than a tubal ligation. I made the choice surprisingly easily, even though I knew it put me at odds with the church's teaching.

The vasectomy itself was simple, merely cutting (surgical

excision) without grafting. I didn't dread it, nor did I bring to it any of the considerations I later brought to my heart surgery. I didn't calculate the long-term effects, but simply drove to the clinic where Doctor Odland performed the outpatient surgery. There were no major complications, though he did take an irritatingly long time with his tying. Within a day or two, all pain and swelling were gone. I regretted the fact that we couldn't have more children, yet I knew we had enough. And neither the idea that I was sterile, nor the idea that I had disobeyed the church (though not God, I hoped) bothered me much, for I felt I had done what was right. It was the first time a medical operation had altered my life.

Last Days

I returned from Detroit with the clock ticking. In a week I would have my bypass. In dark moments, I judged the surgery to be my rendezvous with death.

Ever since I had hid my head under my bedcovers as a young boy, I had vividly sensed that at some point in time I would no longer exist. As young as high school I sorted out the superficial and the serious among my classmates according to who grasped human mortality. As a university student, I criticized every system of thought that didn't acknowledge death's hold on life. I believed that death ultimately makes life a matter of singular irreducible events that cannot be rationally taken apart and explained but only connected by stories and myths.

I always had to fight a notion that my preoccupation with death would be matched by an early one. Surely, I argued, my boundless energy promised a long life. I heartily accepted a friend's comment on my upcoming bypass: I was too big a rascal to be killed off quickly. Instead, God intended to soften me up before he let me go.

The plan my doctor and I had developed was predicated on me "jumping" when I should. He believed it was now time to jump. If things went right, the bypass would give me another fifteen or twenty years of life without heart trouble. When I asked Ted what he would do if he were in my situation, he replied, "Do it. I would believe life had delivered me to this spot. My hour had come." Dr. Kacz encouraged me by pointing out that my cardiologist, James Daniels, had never lost one of his young patients to a bypass. Kacz did concede, however, that such statistics reassure all but the fellow who has to leap.

Cathy stood behind me. She had no premonitions of death —or, if she did, she kept them to herself. I probably would have gone ahead anyway, regardless of what she said. Five years of cardiac discipline had worn me down. I was sick of watching my diet, even though I knew surgery would not relieve me of the burden of being "unhealthily" preoccupied with my weight. My medicine aggravated me. I grew tired of the little brown bottles of nitro that unexpectedly fell on the locker room floor when I took something from my pockets, announcing to the world, "This fellow has heart problems. He's liable to die at any moment." I wearied of the blue and white niacin pills, which, in the large doses I took, caused frequent urination. They forced me to get up three or four times a night and take care at the urinals not to soil my pants, and they punctuated my every car trip with frequent bathroom stops. I often felt I was pissing my way across the countryside.

I was also sick of experiments with medicines. I tried fish oil and garlic pills, both of which brought no improvement and offered far less pleasure than a glass of red wine, or the daily shot of whiskey my grandfather swore by during his last years. Some medicines seemed no better than deadly poisons—beta-blockers sent me to the emergency room twice, having stopped the main pulse of my heart, leaving secondary pulses beating only thirty beats a minute. My slow, gulping, plunging heart, which I heard all too clearly, made rising and falling signals on the EKG unit stationed at my bedside. I was tired of being tethered to my heart condition.

Outward circumstances fed my resignation. I was weary of the college where I worked. The formative and heroic years were over. Newness and experimentation were done with. The parade of second-rate administrators and complaining new faculty had grown long and tedious. Our college—perhaps like the whole business of higher education—was mired in tiresome moralism. Discussion of affirmative action and universal victimization substituted for intellectual fervor and practical action. And there was the nagging reality of increasing mandates with diminished funds. Egotism, self-interest, and eccentric personalities gave a rub to the harness of everyday affairs. I remained stimulated by only a handful of friends who wrote well and were in the majority committed to the rural and regional studies program I directed.

Of course, most of what I saw about old age didn't dispose me to wish for a long life, either. I had seen what my grandparents had lived through, and I was seeing the troubles my mother and my wife's parents were putting up with. To die as my father had—at seventy-seven in an instant—seemed a blessed exit. I frequently teased that if I reached seventy-seven, I would resume smoking, increase drinking, and take up eating almond, cream-filled cannolis. Seventy-seven was a good age for dropping dead.

I associated aging with all sorts of unpleasant things. I remember the pathetic parade of Christmas cards my mother received the year my father died: "Dear Ethel," one of her friends wrote in a wavering hand, "I hope this letter finds you feeling better. I am not so good either. I fell down thirteen times, and now I have to pay." Another friend wrote, "1990 does not go down as a banner year for us. A stroke (for me) requiring carotid artery surgery. . . . [My wife] took a bad fall on the pavement at the local shopping center, resulting in severe facial bruises and a right shoulder hairline fracture." Still another friend, apologizing for not writing for a long while, wrote in her Christmas card, "I've been busy taking Melvin to the doctors and dentist. He can't drive the car. He had the frozen shoulder ailment, and had to go to therapy treatments for fourteen days, three times a week. He had to get new dentures. Today I took him for a bone scan at St. John's Hospital. Next week I have got to take him to Bon Secours Hospital. He has an infected big toe and they have to shoot dye in his leg to see what they can do. He doesn't go to play cards anymore." My mother didn't write back.

On the other hand, I didn't wish to die young. I would miss seeing my children complete that long process of growth that I hoped would return them to the faith and produce grandchildren. Of course, as best as a parent can, I had accepted the notion that they would become what they would, regardless of my expectations. In fact, seeing in their lives my own youth repeated, I was wearying of their false starts, screwy premises, and stupid risks—and I was sickened by intrusions of mass, commercial, and secular cultures into their lives. I found their steps too awkward and perilous to watch closely. Where they trod precariously, I could only pray from a distance, hoping that somehow they would find their way back to faith and family.

I realized that I identified more with past generations than with future ones. I conceded that I couldn't keep up with "my times"—and, in my sane moods, didn't much care. I agreed with the anonymous writer for the *American Scholar,* who writes under the pseudonym Aristides. I too was "Nicely Out of It." I can't remember, except for my last years in high school, ever having a need to be a trendsetter. In fact, when I was young I made it a point not to hum or sing popular songs. I considered them mindless habits like chewing gum. Instead of fashionable best sellers, I cut my teeth on Dostoevsky and Nietzsche.

I even went so far as to believe that an early death was fitting for "the last peasant," which I defined myself to be. I liked eccentric intellectuals who, like myself, identified with a past rural order. None pleased me as much as turn-of-the-century French thinker Charles Péguy. Péguy battled against *fin de siècle* French thinkers who quickly disposed of Christianity but tenaciously clung to their favorite ideology; who lacked faith in the church but believed passionately in the mission of education; who disassociated themselves from the Communion of Saints but passionately enrolled themselves in political parties; who had no spiritual life but a degree, no salvation but a career. Péguy expressed best one of the truths to which my pending bypass had led me about how the depths of adult life are found in childhood—"Everything has been defined before we are twelve."

<hr/>

Each day that I didn't call to cancel the operation, I moved closer to my bypass. As day flowed into day, I felt myself being swept along toward the hour of reckoning.

I had many things to do before the surgery. One of the most difficult was telling my mom about it. From the day I had set the date for my bypass, I had known that she had to be told, but I had delayed as long as I could, assuming that would be best for her and for me.

I knew she would focus on my heart surgery once she was told, to the exclusion of all else in her life. I was all she had left. I was her only son, her only child, and with my dad dead, I was also her guardian and her husband, the person who most cared about and for her. There was no way she could resist drawing a parallel between herself and her close friend, Bee, whose son was dying slowly but surely of stomach cancer. Now, all of a sudden, I might die before him. If that happened, she would pity herself, even though she criticized Bee and all others who pitied themselves.

I feared that my death, if it happened, would devastate her, as my father's death had several years before. Still, I knew she was tough. Five-foot two, she was wiry and exceptionally strong—in my mind, she embodied the lyrics to a popular song: "Five-foot two / Eyes of blue / Oh, the things she can do." She could hit hard, which she proved to me more than once with her wooden mixing spoon. She could pull a knot on a package as tight as anyone, and she could outrun any of my friends until we were twelve. Her gestures were fast and quick, her step not the least bit hesitant. Even though she couldn't balance a bike—in her fifties she rode a three wheeler for a while—she was always on her toes and quick witted. There was nothing sluggish about her. She never wore the aura of the soft, nurturing woman, though she told story after story fostering the past in my mind. She didn't whine. She was life's energy. She was my energy and hope for a long and vital life.

Yet she had been knocked down by life. When my dad died, she at first rallied her energies. She had always responded well in a pinch. She could bear the sight of blood, temporarily keep a lid on her many emotions, put a good face on her situation, and do what she had to do to appear strong. She usually reacted to crises with aplomb and intelligence. The only time I remember her coming unraveled was at my grandfather's funeral. Out of control during the whole service, she fell on the church steps as they carried his body out to the waiting hearse.

At my dad's funeral, in April 1989, she hadn't faltered. She dressed well, welcomed guests in the funeral home, conversed easily, and appeared to be in wonderful control. She maintained her good spirits during the week following his death as we put her affairs in order. We even made her future funeral arrangements: She would be buried next to my father and have the same type of casket.

Her stories blended into her actions. On one gray, cold day a few days after my dad died, we went to the grocery store. Along its entrance side we noticed a man going through one of the store's large trash bins. She told me that he was a beggar who pretended to be blind. He usually begged at the front of another grocery store closer to her house. As we were leaving the store and I saw her fooling with her change purse, I asked her what she was doing. She was going to give the blind man some change. "Even a blind man who can see?" I asked. "Yes, your grandmother Amato said it is always bad luck not to give money to the blind, even if they can see." The blind man who could see responded to my mother's coins by saying, "Have a nice day." She replied, "You are going to freeze your ass off today, Bud!"

She stayed in high spirits when I brought her back to Minnesota for several weeks. At the Twin Cities airport, she threw five dollars in the strikers' basket, professed her union affiliations, and put on a "Get Rid of Lorenzo" pin. The weeks she stayed with us she was chipper. She found an apartment in Marshall in a senior congregate housing unit called Hill Street Place attached to the hospital. She would return in the fall to live there. She went around the city on her own. She visited the senior center, made new friends there, and acted the belle of the ball. She made up a crazy hat strewn with badges and flowers from which, among other things, plastic golf balls trailed. She took to telling folks, "I am a model," which she decoded for them as "I am Amato." When a woman, talking about cards, said she didn't play with men, my mother asked how she had gotten three children.

My friends and neighbors took a liking to Ethel. She was especially flattered when one older fellow, who gave her a box of used fundamentalist religious books for me, took a shine to her. People at the center told me, "Ethel is a card," and remarked how lucky I was to have such a mom. Most of the time I did feel lucky. I had grown accustomed to her highs and lows, her follies and shenanigans over the years, even her impulse to dominate conversations. Nevertheless, at times I resented how much my father, even in death, was victim to her fancies and needs.

One day, on the way home from Hill Street Place, we stopped at Marshall Crazy Days and she bought many copies of a postcard of a dilapidated farmhouse. She mailed copies to each of my children. To Adam, who was to take her to Las Vegas gambling, she said he could own part of it if he would help remodel it. She promised to will it to Tony. She invited a cousin in Wisconsin, whom she considered "a cheapo" (one of her favorite insults), for a long stay in her successful son's home. It was the sort of joke she had always liked to play.

My mother could be remarkably generous, yet at the same time she seemed to need someone to speak badly of. True to form, she acquired a target at the club. She began by calling him "a cheapo" and progressed to stronger insults. She also focused a fair amount of diffuse anger against hospice, which was a way for her to attack Cathy. At times she painfully, even ridiculously, criticized Cathy and me and our children, hurting us all in a variety of ways, making her visits a bittersweet affair.

In Minnesota, she outwardly appeared as vigorous as she

had been for years, but I doubted her ability to return to Detroit and live alone for several months until she would come back to live with us in the fall. I believed she overestimated herself and the support she would receive back in her old neighborhood. But she insisted that she go back to Detroit.

In early August, a month before she was to return to Marshall, she called and told me to come get her. I arrived a few days later to find her a wreck. She was frail, worn, exhausted, and fearful. She had isolated herself. Her sister-in-law, Josephine, who lived across the hall, had done nothing to help her, even though my parents had helped her for a long period before and after her husband's, Jimmy's, recent death. A few neighbors visited her, but neither they nor anyone else could have deflected the onset of a serious depression. I couldn't get her up to pack. She would continually get out of bed only to go back. She, who had been such an energetic packer, who loved to stuff things in small spaces and tie strong knots (a skill she learned from tying bows in a five and dime store), couldn't do a thing. She would pick up an object, forget what to do with it, and then sneak back to bed.

She now emphatically endorsed Aunt Milly's conduct after her husband's death. When Dale died unexpectedly of a heart attack, Milly whole-heartedly plunged into mourning. My mother had criticized her sharply. Milly took up the plaint that life was not worth living and repeated it until she died four years later. Although she didn't dress in black as the old Sicilians did, she echoed my Sicilian grandmother's decade-long lamentation to

God: Why have you given me so much pain and yet been so slow to send death?

My mother had put on a black dress inside. She placed herself at death's door and knocked over and over again. She defended her self-pity against assault with a dangerous temper. She brushed aside my attempts to tell her that she was in a stage of mourning, which would have an end, as if she were sweeping crumbs off a table. Aggressively, she told me to wait my turn, with a tone suggesting that I deserved it. Yet once she cracked, "Self pity—I ought to know it—I wallow in it."

When the mover finally came, two days late, we set out in her car on the 850-mile trip from Detroit to Minnesota. I drove while my mother slept in the back seat. We stopped for meals and spent one night in a motel, where I swam in the pool to get some exercise for the sake of my heart. As far as we went, we did not drive free of my dad's death, her depression, and my heart trouble.

We arrived home as if we had crossed a great desert. Once in our house, she flopped in bed and stayed there for the next two and a half weeks, while I took a planned trip to Europe. Cathy cared for her during the ten days I was gone. My mother got up only to eat. Surely she was hoping never to wake again—to join my father wherever he was.

I returned home from Europe to assume the role of my mother's guardian, and I moved her to her one-bedroom apartment at nearby Hill Street Place. I visited her frequently, and we invited her to our house for weekend meals. She would not visit the senior center, where she had made friends in the spring, despite a lot of good-hearted coaxing by its director and members. She refused to participate in any group activities at Hill Street. She had drawn into herself.

Her depression only slowly lifted thanks to a residually strong character, a good doctor, a new medicine, and patience on our part. However, aside from weekly and holiday visits to our house and trips to the adjoined hospital for suppers, she rarely went out again, claiming that crowds made her sweat and shake, which at times they did. Once a model of vitality, she now told me that age can spell depression, defeat, and so much more that would make a timely heart attack like my father's a special blessing. For most of us, there is no better way off this stage than quickly.

She did make acquaintances with fellow residents and was quite popular with hospital workers, who enjoyed how her banter added spark to the otherwise incombustible bodies and spirits that made up their everyday work. She still had pluck and a kind of bravado. Her wit was still quick enough to keep dullards at a safe distance and to enchant others at first sight: "She's a doll; I'd like to take her home," people said. But her humor retained its aggressive streak. When asked how she was doing, she invariably replied, "Everyone I can." And she was not above trying to shock people. She told her companions at Hill Street that while she and Bee were waiting for a Domino's pizza, they had made a deal: Bee would get the pizza and Ethel would get the pizza man.

⟡

Two days before my operation, I went with trepidation to tell my mother of it. I figured she would at first take the announcement that I was going for surgery with aplomb. She always rallied in the face of difficulty. My death, should it happen, would probably be another matter — but that was beyond my responsibility. I could no more tell her all I felt for and owed her than I could express to my children the love and hopes I had for them. I could pray that God would forgive and would span the gulfs that separate the closest hearts from one another. And I could only hope that my mother and children would forgive what was flawed in me, as I forgave what was flawed in them, and that what was missing in inheritance, twisted in meaning, broken between generations, and left unsaid would be set aright. Prayer is wishing for what can never entirely be among humans, not even between mother and son.

About two days before I left for the hospital, I simply told her at the end of my visit that I was going to have bypass surgery. It had come up quickly as a result of tests and the doctors thought it was necessary. She didn't ask what it was or how dangerous it might be. When I went to say good-bye the day before leaving for the hospital, she knew it was heart surgery. She told me she loved me, and I told her I loved her. I left my mother — my life, my energy, my inheritance, my burden — to have my heart repaired.

Surgery

There were a few people at the university I needed to inform about my visit to the hospital. Not wishing to be an object of curiosity and not wanting to spend my last few days before the operation talking about me and my heart, I swore them to secrecy.

At home, I had to secure my mother's business affairs and prepare my taxes, which made them seem more certain than either life or death. I also wrote farewell letters to my children to be read in the event that I died. I wrote a letter to my wife, telling her that she was the best thing that had ever happened to me. The only thing I asked of her was to say an occasional prayer for me, and, when she missed me, to go cross-country skiing along the solitary trails we had followed for many winters.

In the last few days before my surgery, I continued doing what I always did, even though the world, at least for me, could end soon. Each morning I worked for an hour or two on a book I was writing on the pleasures of golf. Then I taught, read, exercised, and did chores. The day we left for Abbott Northwestern,

I ran errands in the morning, had lunch with my friend Ted, visited my Mom, and went to the priest to receive the sacrament of the sick and dying. After a spaghetti supper, I packed for a ten-day stay in the hospital.

Packing for me had always meant choosing the books I would read during my trips. On this occasion, I didn't take anything I had written. I didn't even consider taking my *Death Book*, a small collection of poems, aphorisms, and reflections on death. I didn't feel I would need such a stimulus to ponder that last act of life. I ended up with an odd collection in my suitcase: a bilingual English-Spanish Bible, to read the holy word and practice a little Spanish, too; a book on Nebraska weeds filled with wonderful pictures to look at in case I couldn't read during my recovery; a collection of contemporary Italian poetry; a small collection of select paragraphs written by Charles Péguy; and I took a World War II book, *If You Survive,* that I had been given in a random book exchange at our history department Christmas party.

With a title nicely fitting my state of mind, *If You Survive* traced one lieutenant's adventures from the beaches and hedgerows of Normandy to the winter battles of the Belgian Ardennes. A war story was compatible with my sense of being embattled and it established a correspondence between my heroism and that of my uncle. I had lately become interested again in the Second World War, largely due to a trip to visit France's cathedrals. At Normandy, I strayed onto the beaches and into the cemeteries and was seized by the scale of death and the sacrifice of youthful innocence. Omaha Beach, where I stayed one night, had been a slaughter bench. This truth seemed witnessed to by every particle of sand and every breaking wave.

If I Survive turned out to be the only book I read before the operation. In a backhanded way, it edified me. Why should I complain of the nearness of death or of what few mental or physical pains I might suffer? I had lived long enough to enjoy much of what was best in life. My pains would be suffered among soft pillows and clean sheets. If I were to die, I would do so under the smiles of generous nurses, while young men of the previous generation (like most of my uncles), whose hearts had not yet beat hot with love, shed their blood on the beaches of Normandy, had their chests impaled on tree branches, or froze to death during the German Christmas counter-offensive of 1944. If I complained, I would dishonor their youthful deaths.

Time accelerated during the last day before our trip to Minneapolis. We started out for Abbott Northwestern about supper time, and by the time we had traveled an hour, snow began to fall. Swirling and turning in ever denser vortices, it blinded us. The snow stuck to the road's surface, making driving increasingly difficult and dangerous.

I insisted on driving. I found control over the steering wheel, the accelerator, and the brake reassuring. Striving to find that fine line between speed and caution, I remained alert. As we approached the Twin Cities, the snow turned to a light rain, and soon the road became merely wet.

Once we got to the hospital, I sought out our accommodations at the hospital's hotel, the Wassie Center. While I felt relieved that the trip was over, I found little comfort in being taken into the embrace of Abbott Northwestern's large hospital complex. I was one of the countless sick of Minnesota, the Dakotas, and other states whose fates funneled them into these walls. The Christmas decorations on the faces of the buildings and strung out along the interior horseshoe drive at the heart of the campus neither cheered nor depressed me. They seemed hung with obligatory care. The lights on the trees hung still in the windless night. The decorations that filled the long matrix of hallways and covered desks and nursing stations did nothing to lighten the oppressive sense I had of the hospital's power. I could not forget what business was transacted here. I smelled death.

I had arrived at Abbott through my own choice, yet I nevertheless felt myself a kind of prisoner captured by the power of science and the promise of Western medicine. My emotions were complex: I had betrayed myself into the hands of the enemy, yet at the same time I felt like a supplicant of powers exceeding mine and a grateful beneficiary of miraculous human accomplishments. I believed that this place could cure my heart. Still, I prayed fervently that those who practiced their precise healing arts within this gigantic enterprise would make no stupid, simple mortal error. I didn't want to leave the hospital in a body bag.

I slept surprisingly well that night. No doubt the drive had exhausted me. I awoke relatively rested. Perhaps it was the good night's sleep that allowed me to respond to my hour with giddiness. Like a soldier waiting long for the attack, I suddenly welcomed the bugle's blast. After a routine blood test early in the morning, a cheery and helpful nurse provided my wife and me with a preview of things to come the next day.

At the beginning of our orientation, the nurse led us into a small room, where we were joined by a very heavy-set older woman and a bright, brown-eyed girl, her daughter, whom I first mistook to be her granddaughter. Almost reflexively, I calculated that the woman's chances, given her condition, were not as good as mine. My prognosis was confirmed when the daughter told us that her mother, who spoke little English, was diabetic. Suddenly ashamed of such calculating, I corrected my confident comparisons with a self-directed sermon that God saves whomever he wishes, and the proud and the well-off, among whom I numbered myself, are not his first choice.

The nurse first showed us two short videos about what to expect during the operation and recovery. The lessons were aimed at patients a generation older than mine. Nevertheless, they were informative, and they did not minimize the operation's seriousness with euphemisms. Next we went over to anesthesiology. There another nurse tested my lung capacity by asking me to gradually suck a blue stopper up to the top of a spirometer. I succeeded after a faulty start.

After that exercise, I met the doctor who would put me under. He was the human point at whose hands I would surrender myself totally to the machines and skills that had made the contemporary hospital a laboratory and center of science for more than half a century. An American of Scottish descent, his bright blue eyes and youthful appearance matched his quick and cheery intelligence. We talked about his career (he assured me that he had been doing this job for many years) and about his father's hope to shoot his age in golf. We then discussed what he would do to me and what the risks were. One complication he mentioned fascinated me. He said some people's mental abilities recovered slowly after surgery due to microscopic debris in the brain. I found the term "microscopic debris" delightfully imprecise. It was another example (like cholesterol filling the tiny arteries of my heart) of how something so small could have such an enormous impact on the quality of our lives. The invasion of such small things, or at least the knowledge of them, seemed a particularly interesting contemporary problem.

From anesthesiology we went to the postoperation room. There we saw two patients in recovery, immobilized on their tables and framed by a jumble of support machinery that included a heart monitor and some bags of blood hung from the wall like Christmas stockings. Both patients looked close to death, especially one fellow, who appeared purple and blue to me. The nurse assured us that the patients couldn't be seen by passersby who traveled the sidewalk just a few feet from the large ground floor windows. I remarked that if I were alive at the operation's end, I would welcome being viewed by an unending parade of passersby. I hoped they would dress in bright colors, carry balloons, and shout, "Amato is still alive!"

This part of the tour proved valuable. I sensed that having seen it beforehand would calm me when I awoke from surgery to find myself tethered to such an array of tubes—a prisoner of contemporary technology. At least I would know that I wasn't necessarily dying. And perhaps it would help my wife and my older daughter from concluding the same. Friends had already warned my daughter that I might look alarmingly gray.

After a quick lunch, we were to meet with my cardiac surgeon, Lyle Joyce. It was fitting that he should be our last meeting. As a heart surgeon, Joyce stood by training, skill, and income at the top of medicine's prestigious and lucrative cardiac kingdom, which, as articulated in the 1970s and '80s, contains in its upper ranks invasive cardiologists, who perform cardiac catheterization and coronary angiography; cardiologists who perform balloon, laser, and other therapeutic catheterization; noninvasive cardiologists who diagnosis, prescribe, and perform stress tests, electrocardiography, echocardiography, and nuclear cardiography; electrophysiologists, who diagnose and treat complex heart rhythms; and preventive cardiologists, who work on rehabilitation, risk factor modification, and disease prevention.

Joyce was a high priest of this medical ceremony. On his table, he would open my chest, stop my heart, cut and sew it, and then, like a priest at mass, where the ritual turns from the passion of bloody sacrifice to the glories of the Resurrection, return me to life. I use this hopeful Catholic imagery in retrospect, but at the time I couldn't help thinking of the Aztec priest at the Pyramid of the Sun. On a high platform with a long obsidian knife, he cut the hearts out of thousands of Mayan subjects and offered them in homage to the ruling plumed-serpent god, Quetzalcoatl.

The cardiac surgeon works at the center of life, the human chest (thorax)—the home of the heart, the lungs, and multiple blood vessels that thread their labyrinthine way through our bodies. He practices his art at the place where blood and breath are joined, at the very seat of life. Yet his craft involves the tools and techniques of the butcher. He saws and hacks bone, muscle, sinew, and flesh. His hands are deep in blood. The royal surgeon of yesteryear hacked and cut away at people with little idea of how to remove the skin or suture vessels. Fewer than two hundred years ago, surgery took place on large wooden tables lit by skylights and torches. The tables stood on floors covered with sawdust and crisscrossed by troughs to capture spilled blood. Only in this century has the hospital become a laboratory, a gathering ground for experts of all sorts, a model of cleanliness and sanitation, and home of our age's most advanced technology, from the X-ray machine and the electrocardiogram to the recently introduced computer axial tomography (CAT) scanners, magnetic resonance imagining (MRI), and positron emission tomography (PET).

Other images of the surgeon convey a practitioner who is intelligent, cunning, inventive, and skillful. The Greek roots of the word "surgery" (*kheir,* hand; *ergon,* work) indicate that he is the master of handcrafts. In times past surgeons used sharp, gleaming, and odd-shaped instruments with ivory and bone handles to probe, cut, and join. Today's surgeons use tools and procedures as sanitary and refined as contemporary science and technology permit. They actually carry on much of their work beyond human sight and touch. They identify their target from all sorts of eerie images and electronic pulses and open and cut with lasers.

I had chosen Lyle Joyce for my heart surgeon simply because

he had been recommended to me by Doctor Odland in Marshall at the time of the discovery of my heart blockage five years before. Odland, who had just had a bypass himself, emphatically said to me, "If you need a bypass, get Joyce. He's the best in the state." Since then I had been singularly attached to Joyce, never considering anyone else.

I wasn't even really surprised when at the conclusion of our long wait for him he failed to show. The same thing had happened five years before when I first learned of my heart trouble. The meeting had never taken place, but Joyce had surprised me with a call to my home one evening a week later. He had looked at my records. He was willing to do my bypass. The conversation was long, candid, and casual, leaving me convinced that when my hour came, I wanted him to be my heart surgeon. What I liked most about him was the buoyant intelligence he radiated. I had come to the age when I believed that grace would be found in light wit rather than heavy sincerity.

I had had a second telephone conversation with him just four or five days preceding our trip to Abbott Northwestern. As if no time had passed between our first and second contacts, he again was casual, unhurried, and straightforward. He spoke as if we were equals. Without reluctance he agreed to the three conditions I set down. Each was important to my sense of control. First, he would do the surgery, not an assistant, as I had experienced too much discomfort while at the University of Michigan's student dental clinic to now trust my old heart to a student's hands. Second, the surgery would not be used to experiment with new techniques or materials. And, third, I would walk out on the operation, even at the doors of the operating room, if at any point I discovered that he wouldn't be performing it.

When I learned that Joyce wouldn't be meeting us, I swallowed my disappointment and didn't respond by getting angry. Somehow I already had come to trust him. I believed that he had a good reason for not showing. I also had the sense that I was deferring to the indispensable surgeon who alone could meet my need. We were told that one of Joyce's colleagues would meet us instead. My wife and I enjoyed talking to Dr. Michael King. He was a gangly fellow with a gentle southern accent who seemed straightforward and relaxed. He provided a second contradiction to my impression of surgeons as intense, egotistic, driven, and high-strung. King explained that equally accomplished surgeons practice their craft differently. He, for instance, attaches his bypasses by sewing around with one suture, while Joyce prefers using two sutures. He also explained that he didn't like to have any emotional attachment to his patient, as one of his unnamed colleagues did. He believed that such emotions got in his way. I hoped that the unnamed colleague he mentioned was Joyce. I wanted a personal relationship with my surgeon. If the surgeon knew me, I reasoned, he wouldn't abandon me. He would try his best. If he liked me, he would not get drunk the night before surgery. Or if he did, he would have an extra cup of coffee before he started that morning. Like my medieval ancestors, I believed that "the saint" has to know you before he will cure you. Besides, it seemed only decent that I should know the man who was going to cut my chest wide open. Furthermore, a person—even if just a superficial image—was easier to grasp than this operation itself, which was an abstract undertaking.

My ideas on saints and surgeons didn't square with much of modern medicine. But I knew that my life would depend on both Joyce's skill and his passion for surgery. He would have to prevent my body from overreacting to the trauma of cutting my chest wide open and stopping my heart and lungs. He and his team would have to guide me across four junctures: when they put me to sleep; when they attached me to the heart-lung machine; when they sutured the new veins and artery to my heart; and when they took me off the machine, so that my heart and lungs, once warmed, would resume activity on their own.

On the table, my life would turn on Joyce's surgical skills. How exactly those skills and God's grace intersected I had no idea. But I could not conceive of making it through the operation without both. I sensed that it was futile to reflect on every possible turn of Joyce's hand, to trust God's concern for each and every heartbeat, or dwell on the consequences of every speck of microscopic dust that might wander into my brain during the operation. The bypass was beyond all save my trust and hope.

⚓

Had I known Joyce better, my trust in him would have been even stronger. The outlines of his biography (which I learned from him only after my surgery) would have elicited my trust, beginning with the fact that he was a farm boy, and I believed that farm children learn a larger variety of skills early on and use their hands more than city children ever do. Joyce, born in 1947, was brought up on an animal farm by a father who served as his own veterinarian. From his early years, Joyce helped his father deliver their newborn animals and autopsy the dead ones. This experience determined his unwavering choice to become a surgeon.

By the time he was a freshman in high school in the small midwestern town of Plainview, Nebraska, Joyce had already decided to be a heart surgeon. He had grown up with the astounding new field of heart surgery, which had begun in the 1950s with the first mechanical valves. The use of synthetic tubing to replace damaged arteries and the development of a successful lung-heart machine made heart surgery a common solution for a variety of congenital and degenerative heart problems in the 1960s. In 1967 the beta-blockers appeared on the commercial market to treat irregular heartbeats and hypertension. In the same year, Doctor René Favaloro of the Cleveland Clinic performed the first bypass by grafting a leg vein to a patient's heart to circumvent clogged arteries. (A mere fifteen years later, 120,000 Americans a year were receiving bypasses.) Far more stunning and most intriguing to the young Joyce were attempts at heart transplants and the use of artificial hearts in the late 1960s.

A high school principal advised Joyce to go south, to one of its few select universities, if he planned to join the best of the new breed of heart surgeons. So one day in the winter of 1964, leaving his dad behind to tend the animals, Joyce and his mother and sister drove south to visit Baylor University in Texas.

Joyce liked the weather and the school, where at that time Michael DeBakey was struggling to perfect the first permanent artificial heart. Nearby, at the Texas Heart Institute, his rival, Denton Cooley, was attempting to do the same.

In 1968, the year when the United States and Europe were politically turned upside down, and the procedure for saphenous vein coronary bypass graft surgery as treatment for angina was published, Joyce, an undergraduate, landed a job in one of DeBakey's laboratories, which was a barn. There Joyce fought to keep alive calves with recently implanted artificial hearts. Despite his efforts, the calves died, one after another. It was the first of two lessons Joyce learned that year about the difficulty of research. The second lesson came when Argentian D. Liotta, with whom Joyce had worked side by side, had a falling out with DeBakey. Cooley invited Liotta to join him at the Texas Heart Institute. Liotta's artificial heart, which had never worked long-term in a calf, succeeded in keeping a man alive long enough for him to undergo a human heart transplant. The acclaim for this feat went to Cooley and Liotta. Dejected and feeling betrayed, DeBakey quit the field he had helped pioneer.

As if his rendezvous with heart surgery were destined, Joyce started his surgical career at the University of Minnesota with the eminent Richard Lillehei. (In 1954, Richard's older brother, C. Walton Lillehei, had shunted a small child's blood to its mother and back, while performing surgery to close a hole in the wall between the child's two pumping chambers.) In the next five years, the younger Lillehei developed surgical techniques for correcting birth heart defects and helped develop the bubble oxygenator (the best heart-lung machine of the era and the precursor to today's pacemaker). Seeing the university's vital case load dropping off, Lillehei sent Joyce off to Salt Lake City, where he could perform all the heart surgeries he needed to perfect his skills. Dr. William DeVries was practicing at that time at the University of Utah. Like Cooley, Liotta, and DeBakey, he was at work on a totally artificial heart.

DeVries invited Joyce to visit a research barn run by Dr. Don Olsen, a biomedical engineer and veterinarian who revolutionized the implant technique. Joyce was dumbfounded. He saw standing before him eight calves kept alive by artificial hearts. The total artificial heart was indeed more than a dream. With Lillehei's unexpected death—he died jogging—Joyce stayed on in Salt Lake as DeVries's assistant surgeon. In that role, Joyce implanted the Jarvik-7, a totally artificial plastic-and-metal heart, in Barney Clark. On the very threshold of death, the sixty-two-year-old retired dentist chose an artificial heart transplant, an operation that, at its best, might result in only a shortly prolonged life and almost certainly would produce a succession of painful medical conditions, not the least of which was being tethered in a life-and-death relationship to a machine the size of a portable television set. Clark lived for 112 days with the eyes of the nation full upon him. Attached to his pneumatic pump, he passed from recovery to crisis, from crisis to recovery, until he finally died as a result of infection.

Later at Abbott Northwestern, Joyce implanted a new and smaller device, the Jarvik 7/70, in Mary Lund, the first woman to receive an artificial heart. He received special permission from the

FDA to use the 7/70. Joyce used it as a bridging device for 41 days until he transplanted Lund with a human heart. She lived for ten months until she died of infection, as had Barney Clark.

Undergoing surgery at Joyce's hand joined me, if only peripherally, to this remarkable history of heart surgery. It placed me among the ranks of all those soldiers, from the Napoleonic wars to the Second World War, whose battle-injured bodies had provided the experimental foundation for modern surgery's advance. Of course, I was also placed among the company of multitudes of stray dogs in Nashville and Baltimore in the 1940s that had been sacrificed to Alfred Blalock's and Vivien Thomas's ground-breaking heart research on wound trauma at Vanderbilt and Johns Hopkins.

Besides his eminent place in the field of heart surgery, Joyce's dedication to his craft would have won my confidence. Excepting his commitment to his family, he is single-mindedly devoted to surgery. He does all the surgeries he can, believing that the more procedures he performs, the better he'll be. He has declined teaching and administrative responsibilities. His true pleasure comes in the operating room. There, totally absorbed in what he is doing, he experiences ecstasy. While his patients are suspended between life and death, Joyce enters a timeless state of complete absorption.

I also found his candor inspiring. He later confided to me that heart patients want mostly to be reassured. Given Americans' confidence in surgeons and patients' vulnerability, surgeons can talk their patients into just about anything. Joyce recognized this as a matter of responsibility. He admitted that it bothers him when one of his patients believes he or she will not make it through an upcoming operation. He believes that the patient's negative beliefs augur badly for recovery. Joyce even thinks that at some subconscious level a patient senses what lies ahead. If this weren't enough to encourage my own superstitious side, Joyce said that each year he becomes more adroit at reading his patients' prognostications in their eyes, bodily gestures, and voices. Joyce also acknowledges suffering his patients' deaths. "They stick with me for several days," he said. "I can't get my mind off them."

<hr>

But on that day before my surgery, when Joyce could not meet with me, I could only trust he was as good as I guessed.

After our visit with his surrogate, the remainder of the day passed quickly. Cathy and I delivered two hundred copies of my most recent book, *The Decline of Rural Minnesota,* to a downtown Minneapolis wholesaler. We then went to St. Paul, where I bought four crosses at an Irish store, one for each of my children. They were St. Bridgette crosses, in imitation of the cross she fashioned out of straw for her nonbelieving father. Perhaps these crosses would remind my children that for me, and possibly for them, the church is a mighty source of hope.

After shopping, we joined our youngest son, Adam, for a broiled walleye meal at a St. Paul restaurant. We listened to Adam talk enthusiastically about his first job at a large computing firm. He seemed launched on a fulfilling career. We had a fine glass of wheat beer, and I hoped that one day we would golf together again—head to head, father and son, on the Irish and

Scottish links.

On returning to the hospital, Cathy and I took another walk through the hospital's empty decorated halls. I read more of *If We Survive*, said a few prayers, and went to bed early. We had to report at 5:15 A.M. to Admissions, which was adjacent to the enormous artificial Christmas tree that stood at the main entrance to the hospital. I didn't think I'd sleep well, but I did—and without any medicine.

As soon as I showed up the next morning, I was put in a hospital gown, given tan booties to wear, and strongly medicated. I sat in the waiting room, entirely oblivious to the surrounding hospital and all the politics, money, science, technology, and personnel that made it run. I was less and less able to focus on the conversation my wife was having with a woman from Wisconsin. Even the blaring television didn't awaken my ire. I only knew there was no going back now. I was too far downstream. I was in the flow of a stiffening current that was carrying me to the cataract that lay ahead.

As they wheeled me to the preoperation room, I teased for an instant with one of the assistants. Would he like to change places with me for money? He replied, how much? At the elevators, I said good-bye to my wife. Woozy, I recall perking up upon first seeing my bright-eyed anesthesiologist in the pre-op room. I joked, "Let's not have any microscopic debris today." Then, at last face to face, I saw Joyce. I found it comforting that he too looked bright and alert.

After he and I exchanged a few pleasantries, nurses shaved my entire body. They pushed me into what seemed a rather open and nondescript operating room. With a little effort and my gown momentarily and embarrassingly opening, I transferred myself from the large cart on which I had entered the room to the long, thin operating table upon which this whole matter would be settled.

Around 8:00 A.M. they adjusted my anesthesia. I was asleep. They began the operation by incising my right leg to harvest a usable vein, and then cutting open my breast to find the mammary artery. They pried open my chest bone, attached me to the heart and lung machine, and packed my heart in ice.

Waking

I awoke to the knowledge that I was alive only to fall quickly back into sleep. I heard my wife and daughter Felice talking in the hall and saw them appear at the foot of my bed. I signaled them to stand closer to each other. I wished to encompass them in a single glance. I had cleared the ditch. It just about noon, and I knew I was alive.

Christ had spared my life another day. I had bypassed death. I had skated the length of the black ice. As I crisscrossed the threshold of consciousness, multiple times I experienced the sheer delight of waking up. Between awakenings, I slept morphine's wonderful sleep. An hour's sleep felt like that of an entire night, which was something I hadn't had in years. I slept and woke, only to sleep again.

With the help of a nurse, I raised my head that afternoon. In the early evening, they removed the deep breathing tubes from my throat. I could talk again, if only in whispers. In the middle of the night, with a nurse's help, I got out of bed. The next morning, my wife found me sitting up in a large, comfortable chair.

According to my charts I was making a normal recovery; in my mind I was miraculously marching back into life. No depression plagued me. No psychological wound opened. I even felt my first post-operative surge of anger as the nurses explained that they were having trouble finding a bed for me in the crowded cardiac ward. I had counted on having a room of my own, as I did for my angiogram five years before, but not even the ability to pay $550 a day for a single could guarantee my solitude.

I feared I would get a TV watcher for a roommate. I wouldn't be able to think, read, or even sleep. Even more, I dreaded that my passage through death's abyss into life would somehow be made banal by Donahue or Oprah, *The Dating Game* or *Wheel of Fortune*. Lazarus would no sooner have been resurrected and unwrapped his rags than he would be sat down to watch a game show. I wanted to rule my room as a survivor of the mortal combat of heart surgery. I wanted to have a book in my hand or a prayer in my heart. Instead, I dreaded that a blaring television set would leach my room — my recovery, my resurrection — of all transcendence. I was already sufficiently recovered to despise the hospital management that had decided that the distraction of television is a necessary part of waiting rooms. They didn't seem to count those of us who are more concerned about getting things straight with God than being entertained by morons who jump up and down at winning a prize.

Fortunately, I did not get the ugly TV-watching roommate I was ready to loathe. Instead, I got a seventy-year-old retired Abbott Northwestern anesthesiologist. He was an ardent golfer, which meant that at the very least he understood that none of us sink all of our putts. His matter-of-fact expression did not deny him a sense of humor. We talked a little about our operations, careers, and even personal traits (especially his habit of not throwing away anything in the expectation that one day his son would joyfully inherit it all). We joked a lot about the excess of Jell-O we expected to eat, but actually didn't get. We laughed until we hurt about our fear that we, with our broken chests, would be enthusiastically embraced by a large-breasted woman. I dreaded being hugged by Marilyn Monroe; he countered with terror of Dolly Parton.

From our windows we looked out at only a few tree tops and a part of the gray skies from which light snow intermittently fell. We did have a full view of the hospital's giant heating system and the great circular pipes that crossed the roof below us. We wondered how such a large heating system could fail to warm our chilly room. During my days in that room I dreaded the chill, fearing I would catch a cold and then would sneeze and cough—which hurt more than anything—until my chest would break in two.

My roommate read a lot. In fact, I ended up giving him my copy of *If We Survive*. His only TV weakness, which didn't appear until Saturday, was football. His interest in the game went back to his days as a successful high school and college quarterback; his collegiate record included a no-loss season. I shared his weakness that Saturday, since my Detroit Lions were playing. Beyond that, I could only slightly fault him for a little snoring and an occasional loud nightly conversation that he carried on with himself. But I figured that a man who reaches seventy is entitled to sleep poorly and argue with himself a little.

Unlike me, he didn't arrive at Station 35, Cardiovascular Telemetry, by choice. Indeed, it took more than it should have taken anybody with a medical background. Only after a weekend of suffering two bouts of terrible angina—severe enough to make him, in his own words, want to "shoot himself rather than endure that kind of pain again"—he sought medical help on Monday. And even then he delivered himself not to an emergency room but to a doctor's office. His doctor put him on a stress machine and in less than a minute promptly sent my roommate off to the hospital for surgery.

Having had his bypass two days before me, he was well along on the way to mending when I got to the ward on Thursday, but his heart was proving to be fickle. Every so often it would stop beating for three or four seconds. Every day a different cardiologist walked into the room and offered a different opinion about this unexpected development. First the staff told him that they would release him on Monday, then that they would keep him a while and install a pacemaker. He met the doctors' changing and contradictory assessments with equanimity. Over those couple of days, my admiration for him grew, as I watched how enviably calm he stood in the face of adversity. He had probably been an excellent quarterback under pressure.

Fortunately, I didn't have to share such worries. Each day

the nurses' and doctors' actions assured me of my progress. I was untethered line by line from the machines and my medications were steadily reduced. After the catheter was removed, I spent twelve hours urinating away the excess of fluids that result from surgery. Stomach tubes were detached the next day, and I was free of the sounds of gurgling and sucking that emanated from the aquarium-like pump that stood at the foot of my bed. A day or so later, I was unhooked from the cardiac monitor that visually registered my heartbeat on a large bank of screens at the nearby nurses' station. Finally all that remained was a single IV in my hand. This plastic tube went directly to my blood and heart.

I also measured my progress by my own actions. By the second day I was up and making solo flights around the perimeter of the circular ward. I kibitzed with the nurses, stuck my nose in their little shelf of books, and weighed myself on a scale, anticipating that I might have lost weight. I hadn't. I visited the older woman who had entered surgery the same day I had and wished her well with her recovery, which, I surmised, was slowed by her diabetes. By the fourth day, my jaunts around the ward and up and down the hospital hallways increased in number and duration and my bodily functions were back in order. I showered myself, washing and drying with particular care the long incision, almost from neck to stomach, down the center of my chest and the equally long incision that ran along the inside of my right leg from ankle to knee.

On one of my tours, I met my bright-eyed Scots anesthesiologist. I told him I was doing well. He seemed pleased with my progress, and I complimented him for not leaving any microscopic debris in my brain. Little things can mean a lot. On another trip, I passed through the cancer ward. The hallways felt shrouded with deathly sickness. Signs with words such as *oncology* (the study of tumors) and *oncogenesis* (the formation of tumors) darkened the pall that hovered over that unit of the hospital. We heart patients certainly have a mortal problem; but the cancer patients—even though many of them recover—have death growing within them.

I thought of my friend Maynard Brass, who had hired me at the college twenty-four years earlier. He was the founder of the history department, and we had built the program together. Together we had fought the wars required to define a new program in a new school. One day, when he was forty-seven, he was diagnosed with cancer after suffering three weeks of indigestion. A quickly arranged operation revealed that the cancer had perforated the lining of his lower intestine. It had escaped and was at large in his body. The doctors at the Mayo Clinic told him that if cancer didn't return in a year, he would probably survive it. The disease returned almost to the day a year later, as if fate had marked these words down on its calendar. Within a matter of three or four months, it killed him. There was no cure, only a short, narrow corridor to death.

His doctors offered him a chance to enter into an experiment testing three different treatments. One of the three—which formed the control group—was no treatment at all; the other two were traditional radiation and a new viral approach. Maynard did not wish to furnish data for science, even though he had an undergraduate engineering degree and was as phil-anthropic a person as I ever knew. He took his solace from St. Paul, who had written of the joy of being elected to the risen Christ. He consoled himself with this message and offered it as consolation to a secretary at our college whose daughter had been brutally murdered that winter.

Maynard starved to death. I remember one day when he was unable to eat the generous lunch he had ordered because of the metallic taste in his mouth. He remarked on the truth of the old peasant saying: "If you don't have your health, you don't have anything." The last time I saw Maynard he was able to suck only the most finely crushed ice. The last demonstrative thing I saw him do, out of frustration and anger, was throw a small, jagged piece of ice he couldn't swallow against his bedroom wall.

At the outset of one of my treks around the hospital, I heard a woman desperately call out, "Help me! Help me!"

"Who? Me?" I replied as I looked over my shoulder for the person she must have been addressing. There was no one else. I scurried over to the nurses' station and informed a nurse, "That patient wants my help." The nurse replied, "Don't pay any attention to her. She wants everybody's help. That's her condition." As I started to ponder the paths that reduce a person to calling out to passing strangers for help, the nurse brusquely brushed by me and entered the patient's room to fluff her pillow.

Later on that same excursion, I met a visitor from rural Wisconsin whose mother had just suffered a heart attack. He was a nervous man of about fifty and fit my stereotype of a rural bachelor, which it turned out he was. With boorish persistence, but not an ounce of malice, he pushed to know details about my operation. The more we talked, the more it became apparent that the Wisconsin bachelor was preoccupied not with my heart but with his own. He told me how much wood he had cut this fall and how far he walked to town, as if he were trying to convince himself of his own good health. Yet in nearly the same breath he admitted that other family members besides his mother had suffered heart attacks. And he mentioned the number of fellow Wisconsinites who had died of heart attacks during deer hunting that fall. Worn out talking to him, I advised him to go for a medical examination and stress test as soon as he could. He said he would.

By the third day, my roommate and I were in rehabilitation. We climbed up and down six stairs, peddled an exercise bike, and took five- or ten-minute walks. I felt confident about my recovery. By walking, I was stepping my way back into life.

If my physical recovery went well, so did my social life at the hospital. My wife was a good companion, as were my daughter, Felice, and my son Adam. I was pleased with the flowers, cards, and calls I received, even though I had done everything I could to avoid the fanfare of the sickbed and the pity and intrusiveness that went with it in our small town and university community. Well wishes came from unexpected sources: friends of my wife, people I didn't know, individuals, and groups. Even the preceding year's political foes sent cards. Despite the pain they had caused me, I wholeheartedly accepted their wishes. I had been taught by my kind-hearted father and by my quick-spirited mother to accept kindness from whatever quarter it came. I was never much for grudges; accepting another's good wishes is part of the command to forgive.

I was truly touched when a few friends from the university stopped in. Dave Monge drove all the way to Abbott Northwestern, just as he had done when I had my angiogram five years earlier. Bill Turgeon, who as much as anyone in the last ten years had, by example and word, taught me to pray, to accept our own limits and God's will, also stopped in. So did Dan Snobl and his son, Scott, my advisee, on their way to a wrestling meet. Dan, a physical therapist who likes outspoken people, and I had struck up a friendship that had grown since my illness. Long-time friend and fellow historian Mike Kopp stopped to visit me twice and helped make a wonderful hospital party on Saturday.

Friday night my daughters, Felice and Ethel, arrived. Felice had bought me a beautiful hickory walking stick. They also brought a video of one of my favorite films, *Memphis Belle*. The movie tells the story of an American crew's last bombing mission over Germany during World War II. Stationed at base amidst the grain-rich fields of southern England, the youthful crew of the plane *Memphis Belle* know that if they return from this, their twenty-fifth mission, they will be sent home to the States. One of the young aviators, caught writing poetry by fellow crew members in advance of the weather-delayed mission, responds to their request to read his poem by disingenuously reading Yeats's "An Irishman Foresees His Death" as if it were his own:

The years to come seemed waste of breath,
A waste of breath the years behind
In balance with this life, this death.

Saturday night, my son Adam brought me an excellent California Merlot. Its richness blended with the warmth of my feelings. He, Cathy, Mike Kopp, and I finished it off during our hour together. The red wine and sweet words warmed my heart.

Nurses also comforted me during my stay. I remember in particular three nurses, each with a distinct personality—Nann, who worried and gave little lectures; Judy, who was quick-witted and liked men to talk about ideas; and Becky, a fellow Italian, who told me about her family and to whom I taught a handful of Italian expressions. They added to my comfort and provided that rare but lovely sense that we all belong to the same human family.

My doctors, of course, won my gratitude but failed to win my affection. I saw Joyce only once after the operation. He, however, agreed to a long conversation in the future, and I believed he would keep his word. (He did, six months later, when I conducted a long interview with him in his office.) One of his associates came by to see me—at least I think that was his purpose. He stayed for less than a minute and never made eye contact. I recall him saying, "Well, you are all right." I replied, "Is that all you have to say?" He said "Yes!" and left.

My cardiologist, James Daniels, never showed up at all, though I thought he had said he would. Each day, at some unpredictable time, one of his colleagues or their surrogates showed up in my room to recite a list of standard questions, to which I gave what became standard answers. They stood at the foot of my bed reading my chart for the first time. They knew nothing of my history, nor did they explain what I might experience in the weeks ahead. They didn't offer any strategies for preserving the integrity of my new bypass. They were as remote as their science.

When I did ask questions, I was referred to the hospital's cardiac literature (which was not very thorough) and to the rehabilitation program, whose two brief meetings offered generic information that could apply equally well to an ill-conditioned eighty-year-old and an energetic fifty-year-old. Perhaps they assumed that part of the explanation I wanted would come from "their new cholesterol man," a doctor who specialized in cholesterol reduction in the younger heart patients. I eventually made an appointment with this doctor for March, when my heart should have "settled down."

From a larger perspective, this neglect was understandable. Who today with any power and expertise is not busy? Isn't a hospital, as medicine itself, a divided kingdom, a place where experts quarrel, accountants dispute, and administrators try to rule? Patients cannot reasonably expect to see their cardiologists regularly, given the latter's work load. Indeed, patients are almost guaranteed disappointment if they seek a personal or even consistent relationship with their heart doctor. The cost of medical expertise forbids it.

I had to admit, too, that the doctors and I had entirely different points of view about my bypass. For me, it was a singular event and a close brush with death. For them, it was one of countless routine bypasses, whose cumulative number in the nation reaches into the millions. I understood why cardiologists and surgeons were too busy to listen to their patients transform their ordinary bypasses into tales of epoch crossings (like *Gilgamesh* and Dante's *Divine Comedy*).

By Monday, my chest began to itch, the hospital halls weren't long enough for a good walk, and I grew tired of living in a shared room. I was ready to leave. I feared that if I didn't make an issue of being discharged before noon, we would be left facing a long drive home in the dark. Just perhaps we would meet on our way back the same swirling snow and icy roads we had met on our way up. I pushed hard and got my way, thanks particularly to help from my nurse, Becky.

I never did see my cardiologist. But I was on the way home—and that was worth a lot. I was filled with joy as I was wheeled downstairs and pushed past the Christmas tree to the exit. There I got out of the wheelchair and gingerly climbed into the back seat of our car, which my wife had furnished with pillows, blankets, and cans of diet pop. Next to me was my new walking stick.

Convalescence

I felt that my convalescence was already under way as we drove out of the Twin Cities, past open fields, stands of oak distinct against the winter snow, and reed-circled marshes, which harbored singing, thriving pockets of life from spring to fall. Each mile home, each hour away from the hospital, made me more confident that my heart had truly been repaired.

With my wife home for the holidays, I had only to tend to my little rituals, which amounted to napping, washing my chest and leg wounds, practicing breathing on the little blue plastic spirometer, doing a little exercise, and making sure every morning I put on my long white support hose, which at first I could do only with my wife's help. Beyond that, I read and started writing again. Each sentence I wrote knotted me back to life.

Within a few days, I doubled and tripled the doctor's recommendation for daily exercise. I began my routine by walking a mile at almost three miles an hour and riding my exercise bike for almost fifteen minutes. I gingerly hoisted my ten-pound weight, practiced bending over and twisting, and practiced short back swings, which would secure my place on the links in a few months. Meantime, each morning I pawed my way through a shoebox of medicines as I sought out my daily dosage of adult aspirin, Lopid (an anti-cholesterol medicine), 500 milligrams of vitamin C, 400 milligrams each of vitamin E and betacarotine, and my large dose of 2,500 milligrams of niacin.

I was convinced that now I would finally drop to my real fighting weight of 165 pounds, which was five to ten pounds over my high school weight. I pictured myself at age seventy free of all medicines, carrying my own clubs eighteen holes a day, and able to bike and walk endlessly. I would be a physical whirlwind.

Thoughts about imminent death were gone. I was tired of concentrated prayer. How many times could I give myself into the hands of God? I now simply gave thanks. I expressed my delight to be alive and hoped that I would meet the obligations that went with it. I knew that I wanted and needed more than I could pray for — and this recognition itself was a prayer.

I experienced moments of joy when everything around me felt immensely light, and my mind was quick and clear. I felt as if I didn't belong to the sticky world of everyday obstacles in which nothing ever gets done easily — not carrying out the garbage, putting a gradual hook on a tie shot, securing world peace, or finding a modicum of harmony at work. I sensed myself free, cut loose from the tightening reins of mortality. I was no longer a man of fifty-five years. I was a boy caddie who could walk and run endless distances. I would write all the books I could imagine.

I envisioned myself skating across life itself. I moved out on the edge of a cutting blade, and with a gentle wind at my back, I effortlessly glided over the ice. I came from nowhere. I had nowhere to go. I was simply the motion that carried me beyond myself.

One sunny day as I stood pumping gas and watching drops of melting snow fall from the top of the pump to the ground, I realized that worlds of recognition can exist in the time it takes a single drop of water to fall but a few feet. Illumination doesn't recognize time or conditions; it jumps ages. Insight conjures worlds quicker than light. A moment of clarity frees a person from a lifetime's assumptions. It forms a timeless moment of renewal.

I was beginning to turn my bypass experiences into finished stories. My wife and I developed a ritual for telling these stories together. We started by taking turns telling our friends and family what the orientation day at the hospital was like. When I told my part of the story, I couldn't resist including the phrase, "And they packed my heart in ice." Then, for shock effect, I added, "They stopped it and salted it."

I also enjoyed repeating the phrase, "I suffered no microscopic debris." If the audience was right, I could go on to discuss my interest in the history of small things like dust. I could explain that Lucretius, in order to preserve a place for freedom in his deterministic universe, postulated that atoms occasionally swerve to conform to human will. Likewise Christians, to preserve the notion of miracles, insist that individual atoms and molecules conform to God's will.

My wife and I took turns describing how the surgical team cut my chest in two and wired me together. We teasingly added that we were unsure whether I'd ever be able to clear airport security.

Also, to show that I was not entirely baffled by the wonder science had performed upon me, I described how they used the mammary artery and a leg vein to bypass my obstructed and occluded cardiac vessels. By describing precisely the operation's cutting and clipping, stitching and sewing, I made it more hideous for the squeamish and assured my claim that I was Lazarus come back from the dead.

I liked attention but not sympathy, so I stressed how little pain I suffered. I conceded that when I coughed and sneezed it hurt a little. But I always was quick to add that I didn't have a right to dramatize my few pains, and quickly changed the subject. I could easily distract my audience by sharing my stunning psychoanalytic discovery: Buried deep within every male is a fear of receiving a Marilyn Monroe–style chest-breaking embrace.

I considered my recovery assured, but on Christmas Eve morning I woke up dizzy. When I finally got downstairs to cycle on my exercise bike, I felt weak. I sat down and took my pulse rate. It had zoomed up to between 140 and 150 beats a minute, approximately twice its resting rate. It was beating faster than it did when I exercised. My heart seemed to be taking off on its own, escaping the cage in which exercise and medicine had so long held it. It was now running through the thick underbrush, beating a savage path toward my death.

Although I was not breathless, which I took to be a good sign, I was anxious. How long would my heart run like this?

My wife took me to the local hospital emergency room, where we were greeted by a nurse. I explained as calmly as I could that I thought my elevated pulse rate to be connected with my recent surgery or possible dehydration. I explained this again to the doctor. He took a blood test of my electrolytes, which I had encouraged. While the nurse tried to calm me and at the same time failed in repeated attempts to secure an IV in my elusive veins, a second nurse repeated the questions the first had just asked. I wanted her and the doctor to shut up and call Abbott Northwestern to find out what to do.

I practiced meditative breathing, I prayed, I tried to relax, but my wily heart beat as it wished. It continued to zoom between 130 and 146 beats per minute. My breathing and blood pressure remained stable. My electrolytes checked out.

The nurses tried to quiet me as the first one repeatedly poked the back of my hand to find the vein for her IV and the second methodically asked standard questions that had nothing to do with my rapid heart beat. Meantime, the doctor was busy elsewhere, and no return call came from Abbott Northwestern.

This emergency was unlike my two earlier crises. Both times before—first in Detroit and then again in Marshall—my heart had beat at abnormally low rates, 36 to 42 beats per minute, because of too much of the calcium blocker Callin in my system. Indeed, the second time the medicine took away my heart's main electric pulse, leaving it going on two secondary pulses alone. In both instances, we immediately guessed that Callin had caused the problem, and once its dosage wore off, my normal heartbeat returned.

This time was different. With my body reclined and my limbs still, my heart continued to pulse madly. No whistle, no command, no prayer would bring it to heel. It was running to the beat of its own devil drummer.

Desperation and anger closed in on me like pincers. I was desperate about my condition and angry at the nurses, the doctor, Abbott Northwestern, and the whole damn business that had brought me through heart surgery only to deliver me to an emergency room where everybody stood around waiting for a call from a phone that didn't ring.

I had challenged the protocol of emergency rooms before. I would have done it again, if I had known what to do. Once, in this very emergency room two decades before, I had ordered a nurse to start treating a burn on my daughter's leg, in spite of her reluctance to do anything until a doctor appeared. Fifteen years ago in Detroit, after waiting for more than an hour for treatment for my five-year-old son, who had a seriously gashed head, I called the doctor and told her that she should take down the hospital's emergency sign. What gave this hospital the right to state in large red letters on its front lawn and above its back door that it had an emergency room when it didn't respond to an emergency?! I won the cheers of other patients who were also helplessly waiting. A hospital security guard soon appeared and kept an eye on me while my son and I waited for treatment.

I kept wondering whether I had had a bypass only to die

because one hospital wouldn't do anything until they got word from another. My pulse momentarily lowered only to shoot back up again. Every time I began to make some headway in calming myself, the nurses upset me. A second nurse started another search for my elusive veins after the first nurse failed. The first nurse tried to calm me by asking personal questions and starting a conversation, which only interrupted my concentration. All the while I could hear the Muzak being piped into the room. I felt as if I couldn't even die amid my own thoughts. I asked them to turn it off. They couldn't.

I kept asking whether Abbott Northwestern had returned our call. They repeatedly answered that it hadn't. I wanted to order everybody—anybody—to do something. As so often happens in crises, I could only order my family members. Reluctantly, Cathy agreed to drive home to get more telephone numbers and the literature Abbott Northwestern had sent home with us. When the nurses were out of the room, I suggested to Cathy that we should call Abbott Northwestern ourselves. Why not call the heart surgeon if the cardiologist isn't returning my call? I asked.

I felt driven to do something. Starting with the premise that one of my medicines had gone haywire, I settled on slow-release niacin as the likely culprit, and I started to drink water. When my wife found a warning in my discharge materials that one of niacin's possible effects was rapid heartbeat, I drank more water, cup after cup. I would flush it out.

The call from Abbott Northwestern finally came through. They advised that I be given a beta-blocker. As far as the emergency doctor was concerned, the crisis was over. I left the emergency room with my heart beating faster than it had in five years, but with a prescription in mind.

Within a few minutes of arriving home, before my wife returned with the beta-blocker, my heart rate had dropped into the 80s. The water had washed out the niacin. I took the beta-blocker anyhow. My wife and I decided not to tell anyone about the episode. Christmas Eve was upon us. Why spoil it with a worrisome story?

I was sick of medical narratives, my own included. I hurt. I felt vulnerable—and isolated and alone with my condition. There was this illness—this cure—this life—this death. I felt like all the old people I knew whose lives circled on an ever shorter tether around their maladies and medicines.

The giddiness of recovery was over with. My confidence was shaken. Evidently I was not to be spared the rub of life's harness. Shortly after the episode at the emergency room, my right leg swelled in the ankle in the area from which they had removed the vein. I feared I would not be able to exercise, and without exercise I would gain weight, be set back in my rehabilitation, and lose what sense of control I had. I also came down with a cold. I dreaded a bout of coughing, which fortunately never came. Pains in my lower back forced me away from my word processor, denying me my primary means of exorcising the demons in my mind. Pains and fears silhouetted my days.

I was afraid of my medicines. Which one, I wondered, was being stored up in my body—steadily poisoning me, laying a snare for another episode? I felt endangered by my cures. I thought of how my dad had distrusted doctors and of a friend's father who frequently pronounced, "Be suspicious while you can."

Even though Kacz and I eventually got the matter of my medicines in order, I knew that I was back in the heart game. I couldn't separate my hopes for a long life from doctors and their diagnoses and prescriptions. I recalled those first days of diagnosed heart trouble, when with trepidation I walked along the banks of the Rio de la Plata in Montevideo. Dodging dog turds, I exercised, meditated, prayed, and repeatedly took my pulse. With each beat, I balanced this life against that death. Nothing had changed.

I knew I had joined all those who live with medical conditions and through episodes as best they can. I suspected that I was in a universe of infinitely small, sinister stuff that had its own ways. Against it I could only hope that prayers counted.

In spite of these worries, my moral compass frequently swung to gratitude. I was blessed to have a God not of abstract thought and a distant universe but of a lowly manger and a wooden cross. I was fortunate to have my wife, mother, children, and good friends. I was blessed with a madness for projects and a keen desire to write. And, now and then, I was blessed with uplifting moments when, free of self, I wished others well in their ways and days.

Christmas Eve passed mildly. I felt enwrapped by grace. The colored lights blinking on our artificial tree and reflecting in windows warmed my heart. A whisper within me promised that I would be around for another earthly season. Cathy was happy. The children were in good spirits. My mother liked the blue recliner we gave her. The turkey and stuffing were substantial. Belgian cookies, made by a neighbor, were a treat. And a bottle of rich red wine was warming.

As a gift, I got a new tennis racquet. Maybe I'd play singles. Cards, baskets of fruit, cakes and cookies—all good wishes given and received are of the grace that saves. I watched the pope bless the people in Vatican Square on Christmas morning, and read Matthew's and Luke's nativity accounts. I thought of Luther's confession: I cannot believe in Christ as I should. He ought to be my true friend and comforter. But the old donkey in me won't have it, and the devil blows the bellows. In my heart it is just as bad as it is in the world.

With convalescence behind and rehabilitation ahead, I believed that on some terms or other I would go on. Perhaps God wanted to soften me more, and further wring the child out of the man. In any case, as long as I had these legs, I would continue to skate—I would still glide across this dark ice.

Rehabilitation

You never return to full health from a bypass. The scars remain as visible on your chest and leg as the memory of the operation is indelibly etched on your mind. Those scars are your Achilles heel for world and self to see . . . and how could you ever forget that you have heart trouble? You are like William James's religious man: marked by a distinct consciousness of your mortality. Only the hope of a successful bypass stood between you and death.

Yet in a more literal sense you truly will experience rehabilitation. You will get out of bed. You will leave the hospital. You will move about again—perhaps better, lots better, than before. You will have sex (maybe at first with trepidation). You will (maybe with even more trepidation) go back to work. Your fear of imminent death will diminish, protrude itself less frequently, abruptly, and largely into your mind. For all intents and purposes you will appear to belong to the order of normal, everyday life. At least, this was my experience.

Surely, I was among the lucky ones. I simply never got depressed—as so many do who undergo bypass or other serious surgery. I did not mourn for myself. I did not feel listless, as if life had been drained out of my body and enthusiasm from my purpose. I wasn't becalmed, nor did I succumb to anxious fidgeting the way depressed people do.

The operation never overturned my confidence in my body. Even though for a few days I felt (to use the words of a fellow bypass patient) like I had gotten the shit kicked out of me in a barroom brawl, I never concluded—or, more correctly, my body never tacitly assumed—that I was a dog without teeth. I started to bite again right away. My essential problem was reining myself in.

Aside from my single Christmas incident with too much niacin, I experienced a quick—if not painless—and trauma-free recovery. I got back to sex regularly, though not heroically. Someone told me (I have forgotten who) that sexual activity would tax my heart as much as climbing two flights of stairs would. I took to teasing my wife about four- and five-flight experiences. And I made a promise to quit counting floors when I scaled the Sears Tower.

Old caddie that I was, I took to walking and light jogging. Walking again proved the best way back to health. If you're up and about, you're not down. I didn't do any cross-country skiing that year, because my chest was still stiff and I thought it might put too large a strain on the pectoral muscles. But I did ice skate regularly. I delighted in all aspects of skating—including passing and outlasting the young. Each strong stride seemed a certain step back into life, each long glide a matter of grace. Being out on my blades moved me back into the flow of things. I enjoyed circling the rink in conversation, especially when I found myself explaining that, yes, I had learned to skate when I was a boy. And "Yes, you're right. I did just have a quadruple bypass this winter. Just before Christmas!"

By the time spring came I was ready for golf season. By then I could swing without restriction or pain. I noted that if conductors live a long life from swinging their batons, I might live long swinging my golf clubs. I loved the shots that proved I was as long off the tee as ever, and with each good shot I relished the boy in me, embracing, to use the words of Emilio De Grazia, "man and boy resonating in the same flesh." I was filled with gratitude to my surgeon and to God and to all others who had given me a chance to reenter the sensual and tantalizing garden of golf.

Out there on the course, with a mind free of everything but the game, I was delighted by small occurrences. One day I thrilled to see a heron take off from the river flats at the eighteenth hole. Another particularly windy day I was ecstatic when six bluebirds circled me as I worked my way up the eleventh hole. Nicknamed "Back-Nine Joe," I embraced my self-definition as a solitary golfer. Alone with the course, I was crowded with the pleasures of being alive.

Such a return to physical activity won me bragging rights. While I didn't make it a point to go looking for attention, and I didn't for all reasons of pride wish to be the recipient of see-through sympathy or even more the object of mere curiosity, I reveled in being told how amazing my recovery was. I took particular delight in hearing an academic political enemy confess that I looked as hale and hearty as ever.

I now had medical stories of my own to swap with others. Bypass gave me license to talk seriously about a contemporary rite of passage. I had been under the knife, my heart had been packed in ice, I had been put on a machine, and I had come back to life. These stories lent me authority. I could even legitimately empathize with those far worse off than me—like an eighteen-year-old student whose heart, if not medicated, raced at 160 beats a minute. He expected he would soon need a transplant.

The very first summer after my bypass I demonstrated my rehabilitation to myself and the world by enrolling on the Tram, a six-day charity bicycle trek across Minnesota, averaging about sixty miles a day. Cycling mainly west to east with prevailing winds, I made the trip with relative ease. I was most bothered at night after biking, when I found it nearly impossible to sleep on the small canvas cot I had brought. And the slamming doors of the twenty or so portable plastic privies—which served the two thousand bikers belonging to our tent city—eventually drove me in search of motels.

The last day of the trek, ascending out of the St. Croix River Valley up into Wisconsin, I declared myself rehabilitated: I had completed a trip I would never have undertaken if I had not had a bypass. I was confident that surgeon Joyce's double-circled stitches would hold. I might even be able to embrace Marilyn Monroe if given a chance. I felt less compulsion to monitor the invisible.

By the time I returned to the university in the fall I was beginning to believe that I was on my way to a long life. Chances seemed good that I would get the extra fifteen or twenty years that a good bypass lasts. During that time, I would be able to teach, write, travel overseas, play a decent game of golf, and maybe even play singles tennis. In the everyday sense of the word, I was rehabilitated. I hadn't died on the table. I had suffered no stroke during or after the operation. I had escaped death by medications. And the operation had not cast me down in body or mind. I shot a few par rounds for nine, bicycled across Minnesota, and scaled the Sears Tower two or three times.

My quick recovery can be accounted for. I was relatively young. I was in overall good health. More than I knew I was an athlete. By temperament I attacked situations. Also, my bypass was elective. It wasn't forced. It didn't come after a heart attack. In some way, I had been preparing myself for bypass for five years before it became necessary. And since I was a boy, I had been grappling with my mortality. I even fostered an awareness of it. I was — perhaps as much as one can be — accustomed to death's hold on my life.

I also had parents who taught me stick-to-it-iveness. My father, with only a little whining, modeled duty and endurance; my mother, with some bluff, taught boldness and straightforward confrontation. Together, they, along with a World War II boyhood, showed me that one does what one can with what one is given. Duty, dignity, and death often conjoin. I had suffered internally for ten terrible years. Christianity had taught me that suffering was the price of life. Besides all that, I was married to a nurse—and it didn't hurt that I had taught for twenty-five years at a university committed to serving the handicapped students who filled our classes. In a word, I was equipped for bypass.

Nevertheless, my bypass was an irreversible operation. It had pinned me to my heart and turned my ear irretrievably toward its beat. My throbbing center—my blood! my oxygen, my energy—was fragile and precarious. If only with the thinnest slice of consciousness, I knew that I was being strangled year by year by the invisibly hardening and closing branches of my heart.

I understood my life as a condition of heart. Let the word *heart* be said, and my ears perked up. Let my glance fall on it in the least significant publication and the oddest context, and my eyes read in earnest. Heart encompassed me as fact and metaphor. It gathered my interest, solicited my thought, bulged my imagination, and made me pray that my heart would beat well forever until I was irreparably destroyed by some other disease. I—like all fellow bypassers—had been solemnly and irrevocably joined to the order of the heart.

Bypass defines a rite of passage. One never annuls it. The surgery ferries one to another bank of life as surely as Charon ferried Greeks of old across the river Lethe to Hades. I now stood on the other shore. I perceived long shadows over life I never saw before. I embraced the dead as companions. Bypass was a long step toward joining my father and reuniting with my grandparents. I was embarking on a trip to meet my grandfather, Antonino, who died so young, and his father, Giuseppe.

And there were others among the dead to meet as well—Phil, Fina, Sam, Milly, Mabel, Aunt May, and many more.

And if this reunion was only wishful thinking on my part, I prayed that it would occur. In any case, I took consolation from Socrates' wonderful notion: Either we die and have the deep and restful sleep age has so long and fitfully denied us, or we awake to meet with the eminent people who have gone before us. Only the veritable presence of God, Jesus, Mary, Abraham, Moses, and all the saints and good souls of the Old and New Testaments could supplement Socrates' garrulous and intelligent heaven.

Outwardly, bypass lay a long scar on my chest. Inwardly, it set death's skull on the desk of my mind. It told me time was preciously scarce, and I must work hard. There is only so much time to achieve one's heart's desires.

At the university, I took pleasure again in teaching and working with students on projects, but I had much less patience with academic folly, though I participated in and perhaps created my fair share of it as I struggled to articulate a regional studies program with the help of a fickle administration, on the one hand, and without the cooperation of the history department on the other. Once known for its solidarity, the history department succumbed to insidious quarreling and just plain nastiness as two of the old workhorses left, and two fresh recruits belonging to a new generation marched off in opposite directions from us and each other. Even though it was not easy to call myself off—I who took things so quickly and strongly to heart and could mobilize so much energy—I struggled to limit and stay on my own property. I learned to economize myself. I simply couldn't rally my heart to the world around me as I once had—not even to defend what I had helped create. I became indifferent to faculty tales of administrative wrongs, and dismissed claims of mistreated faculty to be as common as fleas on a dog.

I had neither energy nor time to fight common problems and reoccurring wrongs. I simply could not parcel out a scarcely allotted life to repetition and redundancy. Deep breathing helped me to stifle those momentary impulses to join the fray that rose up in my breast. Awareness that I only could and should do so much allowed me to still my emotions—the running hounds of the soul. Instructively, I remembered university friends who had spent their best passions chasing the academic swirl of atoms.

Bypass formed a solitary calling. It echoed St. Paul's truth: "We glory in tribulations also: knowing that tribulation worketh patience; and patience experience; and experience hope." It furthered my resolve to work and fused it with my hope as if they were one. In other terms, bypass did what every great storm on the plains does. It deepened in me the rivulets and streams that already cut their way down from the upper margins of the prairie to the valley below.

⌁

Bypass put me in another realm where thinking could not free me or console me: It hooked me to medicine. It tied me— by the strength of all my fears and hopes and a desire to do what was good for myself—to its appointments and lab tests, diagnoses and subscriptions. Medicine reeled me in and out as if I were a fish on its line. At times, I wished to flee as far as I could from all its kind, helpful people. I wanted their sympathy, compassion, and most of all their treatment, but I hated the dependency they afflicted on me. They would cure me; they would—with words and numbers—tell me how I was faring, but in so doing would offer a verdict on how and when I would die.

One therapist in particular proved all too kind. Her attempts to teach me how to relax made me nervous. Her poorly chosen music and supposedly soothing words clanged in my brain like noisy clichés. Her sugar-coated counsel seemed an indoctrination into lifelong fear. I was a fifty-some-year-old lion she was trying to turn into a seventy-five-year-old scaredy cat.

There was also that rank and file of health workers, clad in white, who unceremoniously and routinely delivered my solemn numbers. My life was summed up as a ho-hum report: "Your blood pressure is high: 170 over 92. Your cholesterol is unaltered: 206." They couldn't seem to adjust their language, tone of voice, and gestures to fit the import of these numbers, which, encouraging one time and depressing the next, described my fate.

Every time I went to the clinic I was in a mood, even when I decided I would be in no mood. No matter how nonchalant I tried to be, I found it hard not to react in a place where I felt on stage, where the state of my well-being was routinely announced. This was about me, my future. The mere mention of my weight was weighty business. I remembered the opening lines of the radio detective show *The Fat Man:* "He steps on the scale. Weight: 240 pounds. Fortune: Danger." (I suppose these days "danger" would mean that at that weight the fat man is soon to have a heart attack.) Even when I joked in the doctor's office, I found myself trying to prove my aplomb, my courage.

Once in a while, I even got miffed at my family doctor, Kacz. At times I wished he would treat my condition more aggressively. He would praise me for doing well, especially for exercising, when in fact I wasn't doing well at all, when my blood tests indicated I had come to a standstill on my road to recovery, or I had even slipped back from my ideal blood numbers, my total cholestrol, low-density and high-density cholestrol, and trigylcerides. I understood his strategy. Better to praise his patients for the efforts we've made (at least we haven't gotten fatter) than to criticize us for failing to change our intractable eating habits, which, a friend told me, only change when we get a new job, end or start a marriage, live in a foreign country, or join a monastery. Diet constitutes a way of life, a state of mind, a chemical condition of body—anything but an easily tamed beast.

If the doctor's office doesn't steal a heart patient's innocence about the ease of recovery, insurance will. Sometime after his operation—often during convalescence itself—the bypass patient will discover how deeply the system's hook is set. He will feel himself reeled in by a giant bureaucracy. The catch usually starts innocently enough. The insurance company refuses to pay for this or that part of the operation or rehabilitation, or the hospital continues (as happened to me) to bill and threaten long after it has been paid. All this tests the heart patient's patience and frequently drives him to resort, despite all he has been taught, to old-fashioned, bad-for-your-heart shouting and hollering.

Insurance battles become simple and straightforward cases of "You pay!" "No, you pay!" or, as I personally discovered, they can be vast and complex, part of a whole state's policy and a national debate. Two years after my bypass public employees in southwestern Minnesota got a new regional health provider. Abbott Northwestern, its heart clinic, and my surgeon, Lyle Joyce, were omitted from the list of certified providers. If the need arose, I would have to pay an extra twenty-five hundred dollars a year to go outside the network and return to the people who got me through my first bypass.

From my struggles with insurance I learned with millions of others across the nation that money matters most. I emerged from my battles aware that my medical narrative and those of fellow employees at the university did not count a lot in the epoch's larger tabulations. (One employee was required, until the family lawyer stepped in, to have his children repeat a lengthy battery of allergy tests so they could go to the new system's designated allergist.) Once nature hard-heartedly parceled out our fates; now the medical system determined what it deemed fair treatment. I couldn't afford a protracted and futile battle against my insurance company or the state legislature. I could however, if I had to, pay the difference in premiums. My advantage in this matter—which the poor don't have—was money, reminding me guiltily about the injustice of who suffers and dies, and who survives and thrives.

Of course, the kingdom of medicine involves, as I increasingly discovered, something more serious and deadly than doctors and insurance: Drugs, whose effectiveness is based on the statistical probability of molecular behavior in any given body, can come at a person in many ways. In one person they can erupt in energy, provoking wild reactions; in another, they can lie as still as a well-fed python. However they course in our individual veins, in our imaginations they intertwine with our deepest hopes and fears. They drive even the slow-witted to make sense out of what their bodies say.

As I know, drugs can be lethal. In one instance, the very medicine that promised to help my heart caused it to beat wildly. On two other occasions, the medicine intended to lower my labile blood pressure deactivated two of the three pulses that cause my heart to beat. In effect, any medicine "worth its salt" is dangerous. "Side effects" is the term for both unintended and unwanted results.

As drugs jeopardize the body, so they delude the mind. Desperation sets a person looking for something, anything. The ill person grasps after cures long after he or she has professed despair. Any mention of something good for the heart caught my interest. I experimented with fish oil, soya, garlic pills, and chromium. I never achieved any final proof regarding their efficacy, but at least—I joked with my family—chromium hadn't caused me to sprout bumpers.

The bewitching power of medicine arises out of the illusion

of an easy cure. The great come-on of contemporary medicine is this: I need only take a small and inexpensive (or, at least, insurance-paid) pill regularly, and with no more effort than a swallow I am on my way to being well. I don't need leeches. I don't need electric shocks. Even less do I need to make a pilgrimage or examine my life. I am even exempted from making a tedious daily effort to improve my habits.

In my case, if I take just an aspirin a day—how easy!—my blood will be thinned and I will have far less chance of a heart attack. If I take one of the cholesterol medicines (with which I have continued to experiment with only moderate success), I'll improve my cholesterol levels. And if I take a daily dose of vitamin E, an antioxidant—as I do—less plaque will coat my arteries. Vitamin C might help too, if only to reduce colds, whose common symptoms cardiac patients can mistake for signs of serious illness.

If this were the sum of my pharmaceutical problems, I would do well to simply record a few complaints and then turn around and bow reverently to drugs. But drugs bring—at least they brought me—protracted dilemmas and ambiguous choices. I have been advised by my preventive cardiologist to quit niacin, my favorite drug to battle cholesterol, because it increases my sugar levels. This has become an increasingly important consideration since I was diagnosed a diabetic.

Which brings me to the matter of sugar. I love it. I have always loved sweets. The society I am a part of loves them too. Sweetness may just be innate. It surely is everywhere—and it singularly gratifies and rewards. We even talk of sweet sex. It is found not just in candy, pies, and cakes but in grains, fruits, and drinks. It lurks everywhere, and from childhood on we seek it out and are rewarded by it. As much as anything it is associated with our affections. Sugar, like alcohol, comforts us when we are feeling badly about ourselves, even if it is the reason we are feeling badly in the first place. Nicotine, caffeine, sugar—I have had every one of society's milder addictions. Diabetes, I now concede, has a wicked hold on me.

With the designation of being a diabetic comes a horde of fears, besides more blood tests and experiments with medicine. I ask, as every patient long in rehabilitation must, is there no end to this tedious threatening swirl of diagnosis and experimentation, experimentation and diagnosis? I wonder whether I will die as my father did, weakened in muscle—the heart muscle. In the last year and a half of his life, he—who had been a vigorous walker and worker—could hardly push the pedals on my exercise bike no matter how low we adjusted the tension. Or will I go blind the way one old Italian relative did? I remember one night forty-five years ago when my father, grandmother, and I dropped her off in front of her house. She insisted she could make it in on her own. I watched as she swayed up the side of her driveway toward her back door. She was as blind as the night in which she trod.

Fortunately, my eye examinations were favorable. I still needed glasses only to read—there were no crystals gathering in my eye cells. I went to our local hospital's diabetes center to try a new preventive medicine. The only thing it did for sure was make me urinate with intolerable frequency. I concluded that if this kept up I would end up living in public bathrooms. Every one of my frequent trips between Marshall and Minneapolis would be a tour of toilets. I quit the medicine and vowed — not for the first or even the twenty-first time — to lose weight.

So I returned myself to the principal arena of combat for a healthy heart: diet. But I had no winning strategy. Indeed, I experienced daily defeat, low-grade but abiding guilt, and occasional bouts of self-disgust. Dieting taught me more than meditation ever could about my unruly mind and rampaging body. Snacks, overindulgence, and peccadilloes proved their undeniable hold on me. I could only offer for an excuse that temptation lies everywhere. It inhabits my very body — my individual cells — which ride on the impulses that regularly ply my mind. Food accompanies nearly every social occasion. It is advertised up and down the streets, forms a parade of candy dishes in every office, and is the reason for every menu.

I see the power of the temptation that surrounds and inhabits me embodied in the legions of society's obese. Touchingly sad are the young girls, already too heavy to run or skate. They (at least statistically) are already well along the path to heart disease. On the other extreme are the bulimics and anorexics, while in the middle are those tedious hordes of people who would make discussions of diet their own and everyone else's substance. They apparently never learned that man does not live by talk of food alone. If diet has not become the first moral command of the majority — Thou shalt honor calories above all other matters! — surely it is a necessary imperative in such a rotund society, which swims in fat foods and is tethered in work and recreation to a chair and screen. My heart and its disease belongs to this common morass, created by our unrivaled triumph over scarcity.

For the sake of my heart and our general health, my wife (the general) and I (a faltering corporal) have been engaged in a long campaign against eating poorly. We have tried to be prudent and moderate in pursuit of virtue. We have done more or less what we should, occasionally having meat or pizza or sneaking a homemade blueberry cake or rhubarb pie. (Of course, our sins are more than we dare itemize.) We eat moderate amounts of dairy products. At supper we make sure we have enough vegetables. We use tuna, turkey, and chicken. We cook with olive and sunflower oils. We eat a lot of rice, cooking with a wok. Occasionally we try bean and other vegetarian dishes.

Now and then I read one of those many books dedicated to cooking and eating for a good heart and a long life. Every time I do feel a bit saintly about my eating, I experience a short-lived righteousness. Often I discover I have been mired in sin without knowing it. Recently, I painfully learned that breads (especially my beloved bagels) also turn into sugar in the body. Is there no end to the insidious chemistry of food for us bypassers? Must I do my heart harm every way I turn? Dieting—what sort of final picayune battleground is this for a boy raised on the Second World War?

And again, for me, the matter of sweets surfaces. I have been addicted to them since my first birthday party—or, for that matter, since I first tasted my mother's milk. Usually the sinful apple is in my mouth and halfway down my throat before I realize that once again I have disobeyed the commandment. Quitting smoking seemed easier, at least in retrospect. My darting eyes and grasping hands are wired to the instant circuitry of my craving brain, and my reach is far quicker than my sluggish resolutions and restraining reason. The boy at my center eats, while the man, who commands my reason and common sense, scolds in futility, in the end confessing that his only accomplishment has been limiting the choice of desserts and their size and number of helpings. Sometimes I feel this whole land of milk and honey is organized to kill me, to strangle my heart, the very organ of which I am proud. From time to time I sigh with deep resignation that I should just go ahead and eat a Sicilian cannoli—a cone of almond-spiced cream and sugar—then smoke a cigar, have a glass of scotch—no, two glasses now that I think of it—and drop dead of a delicious heart attack. Better a dead Epicurean than a defeated stoic.

I do justify my momentary slips—a piece of candy here, a dish of "lite" ice cream there. After all, it is not my nibbles that are killing me. It is my fifteen to twenty excess pounds. They send my sugar soaring, coursing up and down my arteries depositing inhibiting sheets of crystals wherever they settle. Oh God, it is terrible: little things do mean a lot. They equal death by increment.

Invariably, when a mood like this is on me, I'll go on to rationalize that if I didn't drink, I would lose ten to fifteen pounds and limit my sugar. I calculate the yearly calories in a beer and a half a day. My math may be flawed though, for I end up figuring that somewhere down the road I will lose so much weight I will vanish altogether! I will be an invisible angel. Yet I don't want to quit having two or three beers with the occasional friend who drops by. Every world-wearied heart needs a celebration now and again.

So exercise is my answer. It helps keep my weight under control. It builds muscle, which burns calories faster than fat does. It uses up excess sugar produced by my body. Furthermore, and perhaps most important, it is something I can do and enjoy. I like to mix forms of exercise: in the winter, the exercise bike and rowing machine in the basement, along with skating and walking; in summer, my ten-speed bike, roller blades, walking, and golf. And there's no harm in walking to work, mowing the lawn, turning over a garden, or cutting a little wood, even if I end up none the thinner for it.

Exercise hinges on walking. It is crucial to having a healthy heart. Yet, here too, I — the old caddie — didn't encounter clear sailing. In this case my Achilles heel proved to be my big toe. It often aches, and a few times it has developed gout, as it did last summer in Sicily. I remember my painful ascent to the temple and the amphitheater at Segesta. And after agonizingly walking the cobbled street of Erice, I sat for over an hour in the front of Frederick the Second's chapel nursing my throbbing right big toe. I massaged it continuously as I imbibed the solemn facade of the chapel.

So my heart leads me to where so many of the old end up: at their feet. This toe, and a recent six-month bout with heel spurs, have ended my jogging. Hereafter I must depend on skating and biking my way back to a youthful weight and health. Getting old means getting run down.

To be a thin boy again is only a dream. At times, I find myself, if only for a moment, envying those who died young, quickly and gloriously. I see now all too clearly how life accumulates upon itself—and how without humor and hope it becomes too heavy for one's spirit to lift. Never live long enough to become oneself.

With notions like this forming the background hum of my consciousness, no wonder I occasionally succumb to a third beer . . . and a second pork chop. Knowledge proves a thin shield against my moods and impulses, and my desire for a good time. As I focus more on my heart, so I focus more on myself. I suppose this impulse is born of being an only and reflective child. It goes hand in hand with my profession as a teacher and writer. It simply joined my insistence on getting at the meaning of things.

My bypass intensifies my sense that I travel alone. It inclines me to be a solitary golfer; it solidifies my preference to skate and bike alone, and, just recently, to take long walks in the nearby river valley. I grow comfortable with myself. My mind scares me less and less. The projects it proposes, if only brief companions for a nine-hole round, a leg of a car trip up to the Twin Cities, or a trudge around the university's empty halls on weekends, amuse me more and more. I am pleased with what I think. I have become—at least some of the time—my own best company.

Solitude—mitigated and buffered by wife and family—now comforts, though in my youth it terrified me. I welcome to consciousness things I can't comprehend, subjects I cannot think through, dilemmas I have no chance of resolving. No longer do I dread loose ends in my thinking. I accept changing opinions and divided resolution as part of the human condition. Save my hope in Christ, doubt is sweet, for it allows me better to explore the world. My mind—willing to entertain more while clinging to less—becomes a more still and certain instrument.

Solitude honed by bypass liberates me from having to worry about others. They must suffer their own constructions of self and world; they must husband their own energies, tell their own stories, and live with or without hope. It is not that I am indifferent to them. I have too many emotions and sentiments for that. Sometimes I feel that praying for everyone is the only earthly thing worth doing. But sickness of heart has taught me that I have but one fate, my own, and it does not exactly coincide with anyone else's. We must each wage our own wars and be blessed by our own light, while casting our hearts freely and large.

Indeed, the bypass has proved a boon. It has blood coursing in my veins, and my enthusiasm has not diminished. Now three and half years later, I anticipate (though never count on) another fifteen years or so. Perhaps I will even one day have another bypass, and another fifteen years.

The bypass has not injured my marriage. Cathy and I still float on a wide and rich river of affection and mutual understanding. Of course, I do not wish to see us older. I wish we were as young and beautiful as we ever were. Husband and wife — at least this is true for Cathy and me — run gently down one sweet and flowing river. There is not much sense talking about the dams and falls we know lie ahead.

A new granddaughter, Rosalia, born to my oldest daughter about a year ago, sticks her head up and becomes part of our world. Like our adopted grandson, Sergei, she extends our love to another generation. Seeing her grow — pushing her in her stroller, teaching her to take people's hats off or kick a ball — provides additional reason to be around. Perhaps Rosalia, Sergei, and other grandchildren to come might find something of worth in knowing me in the flesh as I wish to have known my father's father, Antonino.

The raft of flesh can be frail among the currents of life, but affectionate memories of parents and grandparents, transmitted flesh to flesh, wink to wink, story to story, can prove deep rudders. There is something good about being around. Somebody might need me. I might know the way through a channel they don't. I might be able to lend them a few dollars to tide them over.

Bypass, from which I will continue to recover until I die, moves me further downstream. It has caused me to listen for my heart more carefully. It has strengthened my power to remember and to work. And remember I will; and work I must. There is no other way I could be true to the boy and the peasant in me. Memory is my loyalty. Work, my fidelity. The rest is either illusion to be overcome or grace, so gratefully and sweetly to be received.